DIABETIC GASTROPARESIS DIET COOKBOOK

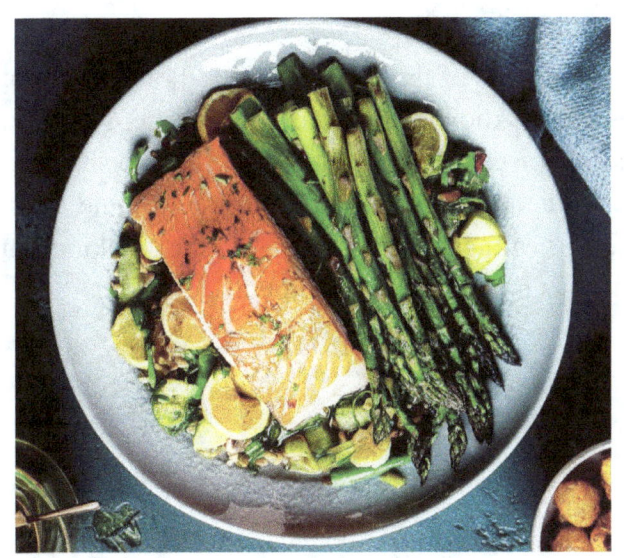

Delicious, Easy-To-Make Low-Sugar and Gut-Friendly Recipes for Managing Diabetes and Gastroparesis

Robert Elliot

Copyright © Robert Elliot (2024)

All rights reserved. No part of this publication may be reproduced, stored in a retrieval system, or transmitted in any form or by any means - electronic, mechanical, photocopying, recording, or otherwise - without the prior written permission of the publisher.

The contents of this book are based on the author's research, knowledge, and experience. They are meant for educational purposes only and should not be taken as medical advice. Readers should consult their healthcare provider before making any changes to their health regimen.

Table of Contents

Introduction..........7

How This Cookbook Can Help You............9

Chapter 1: Understanding Diabetic Gastroparesis............11
    What is Diabetic Gastroparesis (DGP)?..........11
    How Does DGP Develop?............12
    Symptoms of Diabetic Gastroparesis............13
    The Importance of Early Diagnosis............14

Chapter 2: Managing Diabetic Gastroparesis..15
    Importance of a Healthy Diet for DGP............15
    Goals of the Diabetic Gastroparesis Diet........16
    Dietary Strategies for DGP............17
    Working with Your Healthcare Team............18

Chapter 3: Building Your Diabetic Gastroparesis Diet............21
    Food Choices for DGP............21
    Importance of Hydration............22

Chapter 4: Breakfast Recipes............25
    Quinoa Rice and Shine with Pureed Fruit.......26
    Baked Omelet Muffins............28
    Smoothie with Protein Powder............30
    Breakfast Burrito............31

Hot Cereal with Nut Butter............................34
Scrambled Eggs with Spinach and Cheese....36
Stuffed Potato..38
Veggie Scramble..40
Cottage Cheese and Berries...........................42
Cinnamon Apple Oatmeal................................44

Chapter 5: Lunch Recipes..................................47
Vegetable Soup..48
Turkey Sandwich..50
Mushroom Chicken Marsala............................52
Tuna Salad...54
Chia Pudding..56
Salmon with Roasted Asparagus....................58
Egg Salad Lettuce Wraps................................60
Chicken Caesar Lite..62
Hummus Veggie Wrap.....................................64
Gazpacho...66

Chapter 6: Dinner Recipes.................................69
Cauliflower Soup..70
Baked Fish with Lemon and Herbs.................72
Chicken and Vegetable Stir-Fry......................74
Egg Salad with Whole Grain Crackers...........76
Baked Sweet Potato with Cinnamon & Butter.78
Quinoa Salad with Roasted Vegetables..........80
Spaghetti Squash with Marinara Sauce..........82
Delicious Simple Soup....................................84
Zucchini Bake..86

Chicken Noodle..88

Chapter 7: Dessert/Snack Recipes....................91
Almond and Date Energy Balls........................ 92
Celery and Peanut Butter................................94
Greek Yogurt with Berries and Chia Seeds.....95
Greek Yogurt Parfait..97
Berries and Cream..99
Cucumber and Hummus................................ 101
Baked Apples.. 102
Cottage Cheese Fruit Bowl........................... 104
Trail Mix..105
Banana Ice Cream.. 108

Chapter 8: Living Well with Diabetic Gastroparesis.. 111
Tips for Managing Nausea and Vomiting........ 111
Maintaining a Positive Attitude...................... 112
Cooking Hacks and Kitchen Essentials......... 113
Cooking Hacks.. 114

DGP 14-Day Meal Plan....................................... 115

Conclusion..119

Conversion Charts & Measurement Guides... 121

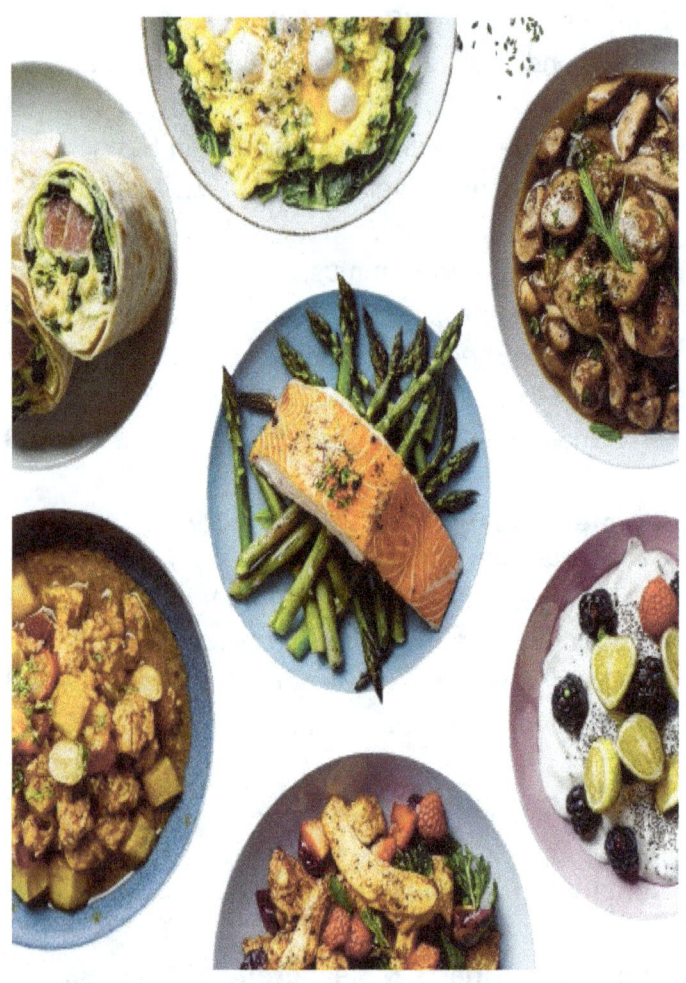

Introduction

Terry wouldn't stop complaining about feeling like a bottomless pit. No matter how much pizza she devoured, that gnawing emptiness hung around. We joked it was her mutant power – inhale endless slices, never gain a pound. But the laughter died fast when the doc hit us with the diagnosis: diabetic gastroparesis. Boom. Pizza went from superpower to punishment. Food, the stuff that fueled our late-night talks and weekend brunches, turned into the enemy. Terry's usual spark dimmed, replaced by constant nausea and a frustration that aged her years. It was like watching a butterfly with clipped wings.

As a doctor, I knew meds could help some, but this nagging feeling wouldn't quit. Food is more than just calories and macros, it's the glue that holds our social lives together. It's the tradition that connects cultures, the warm hug in a bowl that fills your belly and makes you smile. It's the centerpiece of celebrations, the reason friends gather around plates piled high with deliciousness. Terry deserved all that good stuff again.

That's when the lightbulb went off. What if we could turn food back into Terry's friend, not her foe? We embarked on a full-on food mission, a quest for yummy meals that wouldn't declare war on her stomach. We deep-dived cookbooks, scoured the internet for inspiration, and even braved the unfamiliar aisles of the grocery store (hello, weird new ingredients!). We researched, we experimented, and most importantly, we taste-tested like crazy. It wasn't just about getting nutrients in her, it was about rediscovering the explosion of flavors and textures that food can be.

Slowly, things started to change. Smoothies became her energizing breakfast, a kick-start to her day that tasted like sunshine in a glass. Puréed soups, once a reminder of limitations, became comforting lunches packed with unexpected flavor bombs. And yes, there were even soft, melt-in-your-mouth desserts that didn't leave her feeling like a ticking time bomb. Bite by delicious bite, a smile found its way back to Terry's face. Food wasn't the enemy anymore, it was the bridge back to her life.

This book isn't just a recipe collection for people with diabetic gastroparesis. It's about reclaiming the joy of eating, one delicious bite at a time. It's about proving that even with challenges, there's a path to a vibrant, flavorful life. It's a reminder that even when life throws curveballs, there's always a way to find comfort, joy, and connection – sometimes, in the most unexpected places, like a perfectly blended smoothie or a bowl of creamy soup that warms your soul from the inside out.

How This Cookbook Can Help You

This "Diabetic Gastroparesis Diet Cookbook" is designed to be your partner in navigating this challenge. Here's what you can expect:

- **Clear Explanations**: We'll break down the basics of DGP, its connection to diabetes, and how diet plays a vital role in managing symptoms.
- **Dietary Guidance**: Discover a range of delicious and nutritious food options specifically chosen for their ease of digestion. From refreshing smoothies to comforting soups, we'll guide you towards building a healthy and enjoyable diabetic gastroparesis diet.
- **Meal Planning Made Easy**: Sample meal plans offer a framework to get you started, while recipe chapters provide inspiration and variety for breakfast, lunch, dinner, and even snacks.
- **Bonus Chapter on Living Well**: We understand that DGP goes beyond just food. This bonus chapter explores strategies for managing nausea and vomiting, maintaining a positive attitude, and finding the right resources for support.

This cookbook is a resource to empower you on your journey towards managing diabetic gastroparesis. With the right knowledge and delicious recipes at your fingertips, you can navigate this new challenge and maintain a healthy and fulfilling life.

Chapter 1: Understanding Diabetic Gastroparesis

Diabetic gastroparesis (DGP) can be a confusing and frustrating condition. This chapter aims to shed light on what DGP is, how it develops in relation to diabetes, and the symptoms you might experience. By understanding DGP, you can be better equipped to manage it and improve your overall well-being.

What is Diabetic Gastroparesis (DGP)?

Imagine your stomach as a muscular food processor, breaking down what you eat for proper digestion. In healthy digestion, the stomach muscles contract rhythmically, churning and pushing food into the small intestine for further processing.

However, in gastroparesis, the nerves and muscles in your stomach malfunction. This disrupts the normal process, causing food to move through your digestive system much slower than usual. This can lead to a variety of uncomfortable symptoms, and in the case of diabetic gastroparesis (DGP), it's often linked to nerve damage caused by high blood sugar levels.

How Does DGP Develop?

Your gut feeling isn't so far off! Your nerves actually play a super important role in breaking down your food. It sends signals to the muscles in your stomach wall, telling them to contract and move food along. In DGP, these signals become disrupted. This disruption can have several causes, but in the case of diabetic gastroparesis, the culprit is often chronic high blood sugar levels.

Over time, poorly controlled diabetes can damage nerves throughout the body, including those that control your stomach. This damage can lead to:

- **Weakened stomach muscles**: The muscles in your stomach wall may not contract as forcefully, hindering the proper breakdown and movement of food.
- **Delayed stomach emptying**: Food stays in your stomach for a longer time than usual, leading to feelings of fullness, nausea, and discomfort.
- **Nerve signal problems**: The signals sent by your nervous system to your stomach muscles become less coordinated, further disrupting the digestive process.

It's important to note that DGP isn't exclusive to diabetes. It can also occur due to viral infections, certain surgeries, or other medical conditions. However, diabetes remains the most common cause of gastroparesis.

Symptoms of Diabetic Gastroparesis

The symptoms of DGP can vary from person to person, and sometimes they can be mild and easily dismissed. But heads up, there are some warning signs to be on the lookout for:

- **Nausea and vomiting**: This is often the most prominent symptom, with food sitting in your stomach for extended periods leading to nausea and the urge to vomit.
- **Feeling full after eating very little**: Even small portions of food can cause a feeling of fullness or bloating due to the slow emptying of your stomach.
- **Loss of appetite**: The discomfort associated with DGP can lead to a decreased desire to eat.
- **Upper abdominal pain**: Discomfort or pain in the upper part of your abdomen can be a symptom of DGP.

- **Weight loss**: Difficulty eating and the inability to absorb nutrients from food can lead to unintended weight loss.

The Importance of Early Diagnosis

If you're feeling any of the aforementioned symptoms, it's crucial to seek medical attention. Early diagnosis and management of DGP can significantly improve your quality of life and prevent potential complications.

The next chapter will examine the management of DGP and explore how diet can play a pivotal role in its management.

Chapter 2: Managing Diabetic Gastroparesis

Diabetic gastroparesis (DGP) can be a challenging condition, but with proper management, you can effectively control your symptoms and maintain a healthy lifestyle. This chapter explores the importance of diet in managing DGP, outlines the goals of a diabetic gastroparesis diet, and highlights other treatment options you might consider in collaboration with your healthcare team.

Importance of a Healthy Diet for DGP

While there's no cure for DGP, dietary modifications play a crucial role in managing its symptoms. The right foods can significantly improve your digestion, reduce discomfort, and ensure you receive the nutrients your body needs. Here's how a healthy diabetic gastroparesis diet benefits you:

- **Promotes Faster Digestion**: By focusing on easily digestible foods, you can minimize the time food spends in your stomach, reducing nausea, vomiting, and feelings of fullness.

- **Maintains Blood Sugar Levels**: Choosing foods that are low in sugar and fat helps you manage your diabetes, which in turn can improve nerve function and potentially benefit your stomach muscles.
- **Prevents Dehydration**: DGP can sometimes lead to dehydration due to frequent vomiting or difficulty absorbing fluids. A well-balanced diet with adequate hydration is essential.
- **Provides Essential Nutrients**: DGP can make it difficult to absorb nutrients from food. Including a variety of nutrient-rich foods ensures your body gets the vitamins and minerals it needs.

Goals of the Diabetic Gastroparesis Diet

The primary goal of the diabetic gastroparesis diet is to:

- **Minimize symptoms**: Reduce nausea, vomiting, and feelings of fullness by focusing on easily digestible foods and smaller, more frequent meals.
- **Maintain good blood sugar control**: Manage your diabetes to potentially improve nerve function and overall well-being.

- **Prevent dehydration**: Ensure adequate fluid intake to prevent complications.
- **Maintain a healthy weight**: Nutrient-dense foods can help you maintain a healthy weight despite potential challenges with eating.

Dietary Strategies for DGP

Here are some key dietary strategies to incorporate into your diabetic gastroparesis diet:

- **Focus on Liquids and Soft Foods**: Liquids and well-blended or puréed foods are easier for your stomach to digest. Your tummy will thank you for slurping down smoothies, soups, and mashed veggies!
- **Choose Low-Fiber Foods**: High-fiber foods take longer to digest, which can worsen symptoms. Opt for refined grains, well-cooked vegetables, and fruits without skin.
- **Eat Smaller, More Frequent Meals**: Distribute your daily food intake into smaller meals and snacks throughout the day. This reduces the workload on your stomach and helps manage symptoms.

- **Chew Thoroughly**: Chomping your food into tiny bits helps your stomach do its job way easier.
- **Stay Hydrated**: Drink plenty of fluids throughout the day, including water, clear broths, and sugar-free sports drinks.
- **Limit Foods that Slow Digestion**: Avoid fatty, greasy, and fried foods, as they can take longer to digest and exacerbate symptoms.
- **Minimize Sugary Drinks**: Opt for water or unsweetened beverages. Sugary drinks can raise blood sugar levels and worsen gastroparesis symptoms.

Working with Your Healthcare Team

A crucial aspect of managing DGP is collaborating with your healthcare team. They can help you develop a personalized diabetic gastroparesis diet plan that caters to your specific needs and preferences. Here's what to expect:

- **Nutritional Consultation**: A registered dietitian can guide you on food choices, portion sizes, and meal planning strategies to manage DGP effectively.

- **Medication Management**: Medications might be prescribed to help stimulate stomach muscle contractions and improve digestion.
- **Other Treatment Options**: In some cases, your doctor might recommend additional interventions like gastric electrical stimulation or feeding tubes to ensure adequate nutrition and hydration.

Remember, managing DGP requires a multi-pronged approach. By following a well-planned diet, collaborating with your healthcare team, and potentially incorporating other treatment options, you can effectively manage your symptoms and live a healthy and fulfilling life.

The next chapter will delve deeper into building a diabetic gastroparesis diet, providing you with specific food choices, sample meal plans, and the importance of staying hydrated.

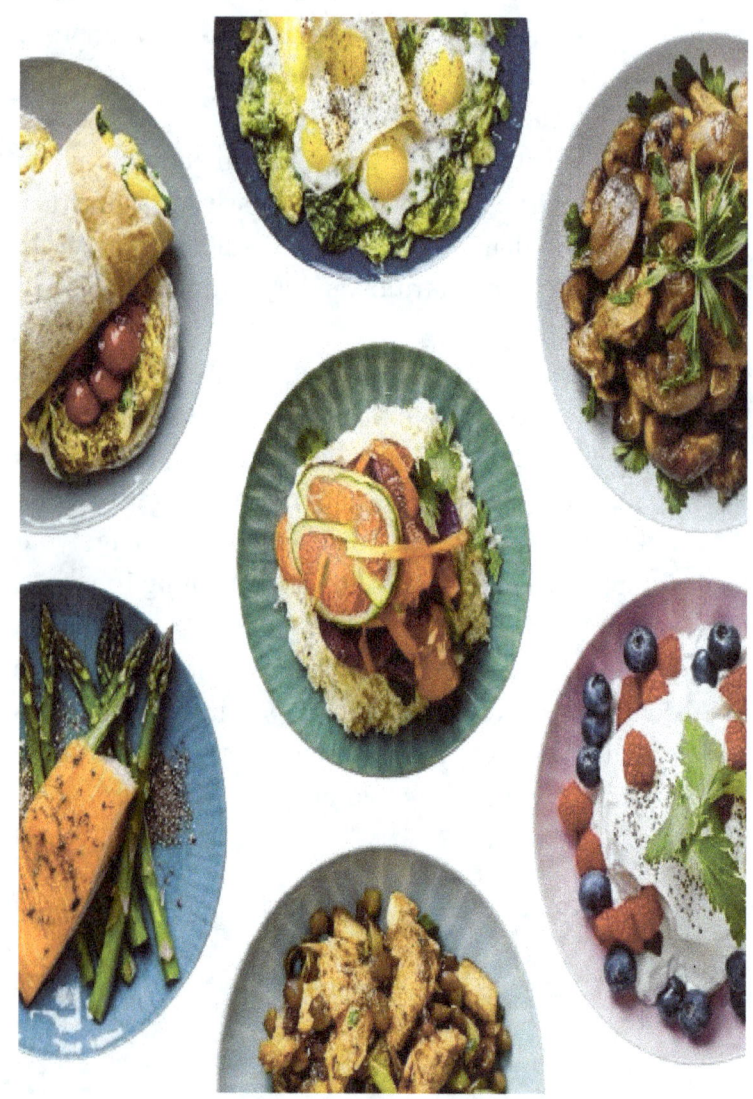

Chapter 3: Building Your Diabetic Gastroparesis Diet

Living with diabetic gastroparesis (DGP) requires making adjustments to your diet. This chapter equips you with the knowledge and tools to build a personalized diabetic gastroparesis diet that promotes healthy digestion, manages your blood sugar, and keeps you feeling your best.

Food Choices for DGP

The key to managing DGP through diet lies in choosing foods that are easy for your stomach to digest and absorb. Let's break it down into key areas to focus on:

1. Liquids and Smoothies: Liquids are readily absorbed and put minimal strain on your digestive system. Consider incorporating:
- **Water (essential for hydration)**
- **Clear broths (vegetable or chicken)**
- **Sugar-free protein shakes**
- **Smoothies made with low-fiber fruits (bananas, mangoes), yogurt, and low-fat milk**

2. Soft and Easily Digestible Foods: Opt for well-cooked, mashed, or puréed versions of these foods:
- **Fruits**: Canned peaches, applesauce, ripe bananas, melons
- **Vegetables**: Well-cooked potatoes, carrots, green beans, spinach (blended)
- **Proteins**: Skinless, lean chicken or fish, soft-cooked eggs, tofu (blended)
- **Grains**: White rice, white bread, cream of wheat, refined cereals (check fiber content)

Importance of Hydration

Staying hydrated is crucial for everyone, but even more so for those with DGP. Frequent vomiting and difficulty absorbing fluids can lead to dehydration. Here's the lowdown on staying hydrated like a boss:

- Drink plenty of water throughout the day, aiming for eight glasses or more.
- Include clear broths and sugar-free sports drinks in your fluid intake.
- Add slices of lemon, cucumber, or berries to water for a refreshing twist.
- Consider incorporating ice chips or popsicles if tolerated.

Additional Tips:
- **Eat Slowly and Chew Thoroughly**: This allows your body to start breaking down food in your mouth, easing the workload on your stomach.
- **Listen to Your Body**: Pay attention to how you feel after eating certain foods. If something seems to worsen your symptoms, avoid it or adjust the portion size.
- **Experiment with Flavors**: While focusing on easily digestible foods, don't be afraid to experiment with herbs, spices, and low-sugar seasonings to keep your meals enjoyable.

The Road to Success

Building a diabetic gastroparesis diet requires some experimentation and adjustments. However, with the knowledge and resources provided in this chapter, you have a strong foundation to create a personalized plan that promotes healthy digestion, maintains good blood sugar control, and helps you manage your DGP effectively.

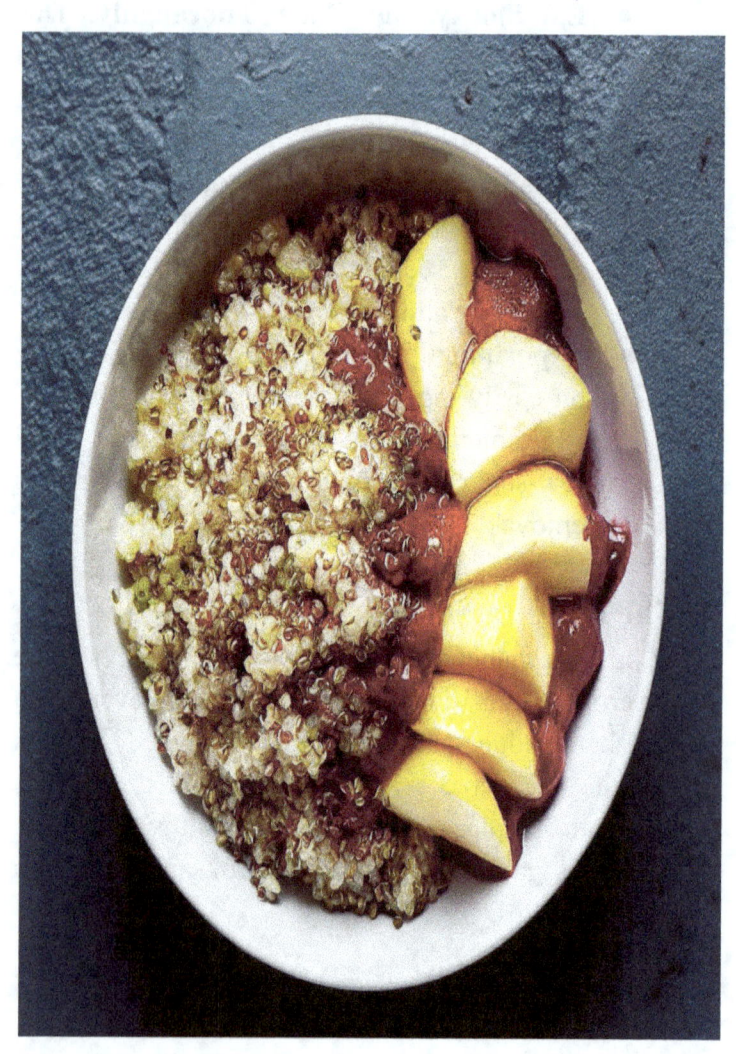

Chapter 4: Breakfast Recipes

Quinoa Rice and Shine with Pureed Fruit
Baked Omelet Muffins
Smoothie with Protein Powder
Breakfast Burrito
Hot Cereal with Nut Butter
Scrambled Eggs with Spinach and Cheese
Stuffed Potato
Veggie Scramble
Cottage Cheese and Berries
Cinnamon Apple Oatmeal

Quinoa Rice and Shine with Pureed Fruit

A nutritious, easy-to-digest breakfast option that combines the health benefits of quinoa and rice with the natural sweetness of fruit, tailored for diabetic gastroparesis management.

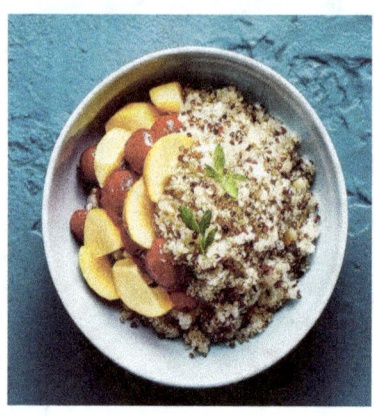

Preparation Time: 10 minutes
Cooking Time: 20 minutes
Servings: 2

Ingredients:
- 1/4 cup quinoa, rinsed
- 1/4 cup white rice
- 1 cup water
- 1/2 cup low-fat milk or almond milk
- 1/2 cup pureed fruit (such as banana or cooked apple)
- Cinnamon to taste (optional)

Directions:
1. Combine quinoa, rice, and water in a medium saucepan. Bring to a boil.
2. Reduce heat to low, cover, and simmer until the grains are tender and the water is absorbed, about 20 minutes.
3. Stir in milk and simmer for another 5 minutes until creamy.
4. Let cool slightly, then stir in the pureed fruit and cinnamon (if using).
5. Serve warm for a comforting breakfast.

Nutritional Value Per Serving:
Calories: 220 | Carbs: 45g | Fiber: 3g | Protein: 6g | Sodium: 30mg | Sugar: 8g

---

Tips and Substitutions:
- Use any tolerated pureed fruit for variety.
- For those who need less fiber, using white rice alone is an option.

Baked Omelet Muffins

These protein-packed omelet muffins are customizable, easy to digest, and perfect for a nutritious breakfast or snack, suitable for people managing diabetes and gastroparesis.

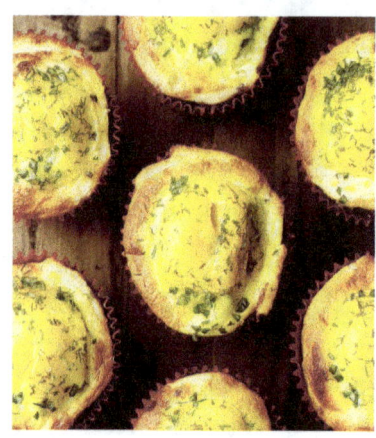

Preparation Time: 15 minutes
Cooking Time: 20 minutes
Servings: 6 muffins

Ingredients:
- 4 eggs
- 1/4 cup low-fat milk
- 1/2 cup cooked and finely chopped spinach (water squeezed out)
- 1/4 cup grated cheddar cheese (low-fat, if preferred)
- Salt and pepper to taste

Directions:
1. Preheat the oven to 350°F (175°C) and lightly grease a 6-cup muffin pan.
2. In a bowl, whisk together eggs and milk until smooth.
3. Stir in the spinach and cheddar cheese. Season with salt and pepper.
4. Divide the mixture evenly among the muffin cups.
5. Bake for 20 minutes, or until the eggs are set and lightly golden on top.
6. Let cool for a few minutes before removing from the pan.

Nutritional Value Per Serving:
Calories: 100 | Carbs: 2g | Fiber: 0.5g | Protein: 8g | Sodium: 150mg | Sugar: 1g

---

Tips and Substitutions:
- Egg whites can be used instead of whole eggs for lower fat content.
- Feel free to substitute spinach with any tolerated, cooked vegetables.

Smoothie with Protein Powder

A versatile and quick smoothie that packs protein and essential nutrients, easily adaptable to any dietary restrictions related to diabetic gastroparesis.

Preparation Time: 5 minutes
Cooking Time: 0 minutes
Servings: 1

Ingredients:
- 1 cup creamy almond milk (or any other low-fat milk)
- 1/2 banana or 1/2 cup tolerated canned fruit
- 1 scoop protein powder (whey or plant-based, unsweetened)
- Ice cubes (optional)

Directions:
1. Combine all ingredients in a blender.
2. Blend on high speed until smooth.
3. Adjust thickness by adding more milk or ice, as preferred.
4. Serve immediately.

Nutritional Value Per Serving:
Calories: 200 | Carbs: 20g | Fiber: 2g |
Protein: 20g | Sodium: 170mg | Sugar: 10g

Tips and Substitutions:
- Choose a protein powder that is low in sugar and suitable for diabetics.
- If you have a hard time digesting raw fruits, canned fruits in juice (not syrup) can be a gentler option.

Breakfast Burrito

A gentle yet satisfying breakfast option that wraps scrambled eggs and tolerated vegetables in a soft tortilla, making it a customizable choice for those with diabetic gastroparesis.

Preparation Time: 10 minutes
Cooking Time: 5 minutes
Servings: 1

Ingredients:
- 1 large egg (or 2 egg whites), beaten
- 1 low-carb, soft flour tortilla
- 1/4 cup cooked, shredded chicken (optional)
- 1/4 cup grated low-fat cheese
- 1/4 cup well-cooked spinach
- Salt and pepper to taste

Directions:
1. Scramble the egg in a non-stick skillet over medium heat until fully cooked. Season with salt and pepper.
2. Warm the tortilla in the microwave for 10 seconds to make it pliable.
3. On the tortilla, layer the scrambled egg, chicken (if using), cheese, and spinach.

4. Roll up the tortilla, folding in the sides to enclose the filling.

5. Serve immediately or wrap in foil to keep warm.

Nutritional Value Per Serving:
Calories: 250 (with chicken) | Carbs: 18g Fiber: 1g | Protein: 20g | Sodium: 400mg | Sugar: 2g

---

Tips and Substitutions:
- Substitute chicken with any tolerated protein.
- For a softer filling, ensure vegetables are well-cooked.
- Use a gluten-free tortilla if needed.

Hot Cereal with Nut Butter

A warm, comforting cereal that's easy to digest and fortified with nut butter for added protein and flavor, designed for those managing diabetes and gastroparesis.

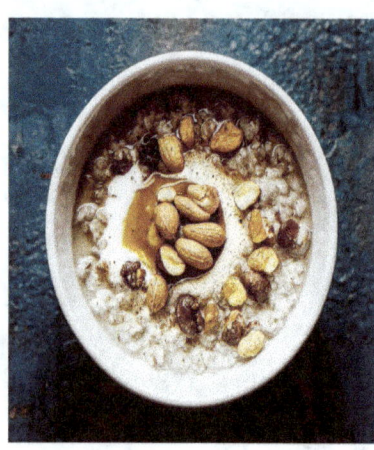

Preparation Time: 5 minutes
Cooking Time: 5 minutes
Servings: 1

Ingredients:
- 1/2 cup quick-cooking oats or cream of wheat
- 1 cup water or low-fat milk
- 1 tablespoon smooth nut butter (almond or peanut)
- Cinnamon to taste (optional)
- 1 teaspoon of honey or maple syrup (skip it if you want to keep it sugar-free!)

Directions:
1. Cook oats or cream of wheat according to package instructions using water or milk.
2. Once cooked, stir in the nut butter until well combined.
3. Add cinnamon and honey or maple syrup if desired.
4. Serve warm.

Nutritional Value Per Serving:
Calories: 200 | Carbs: 27g | Fiber: 4g | Protein: 7g | Sodium: 100mg | Sugar: 3g (without added sweetener)

Tips and Substitutions:
- Use any tolerated nut or seed butter.
- For those who need a gluten-free option, ensure oats are certified gluten-free or opt for cream of rice.

Scrambled Eggs with Spinach and Cheese

Simple yet nutritious, this meal combines the protein from eggs with the mild flavors of spinach and cheese, suitable for a gastroparesis-friendly diet.

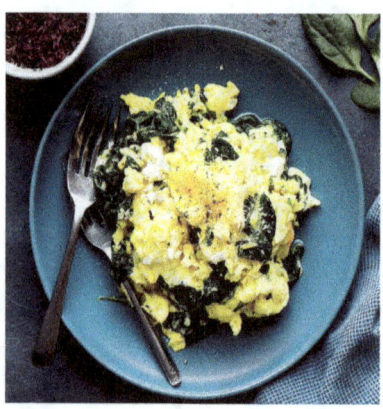

Preparation Time: 5 minutes
Cooking Time: 5 minutes
Servings: 1

Ingredients:
- 2 eggs
- 1/4 cup cooked spinach, water pressed out
- 1/4 cup grated low-fat cheese
- Salt and pepper to taste

Directions:
1. Beat the eggs in a bowl. Season with salt and pepper.

2. Cook the eggs in a non-stick skillet over medium heat until they begin to set.
3. Add the spinach and cheese. Continue to cook, stirring until the eggs are fully cooked and the cheese is melted.
4. Serve hot.

Nutritional Value Per Serving:
Calories: 220 | Carbs: 2g | Fiber: 1g |
Protein: 18g | Sodium: 390mg | Sugar: 1g

Tips and Substitutions:
- Egg whites can be used for a lower-fat option.
- Any tolerated, well-cooked vegetable can be substituted for spinach.

Stuffed Potato

A versatile and satisfying dish, featuring a baked potato stuffed with a mix of tolerated protein and vegetables, perfect for a nutrient-rich meal.

Preparation Time: 10 minutes (plus baking time)
Cooking Time: 1 hour
Servings: 1

Ingredients:
- 1 large russet potato
- 1/4 cup cooked chicken, shredded
- 1/4 cup well-cooked broccoli, chopped
- 1/4 cup grated low-fat cheese
- Salt and pepper to taste

Directions:
1. Preheat oven to 400°F (200°C). Prick the potato several times with a fork and bake until tender, about 1 hour.
2. Once the potato is cool enough to handle, cut it open and fluff the inside with a fork.
3. Mix the chicken and broccoli with half of the cheese; season with salt and pepper. Stuff this mixture into the potato.
4. Top the stuffed potato with the remaining cheese.

5. Return the potato to the oven or microwave until the cheese is melted.
6. Serve warm.

Nutritional Value Per Serving:
Calories: 300 | Carbs: 37g | Fiber: 4g | Protein: 18g | Sodium: 200mg | Sugar: 2g

---

Tips and Substitutions:
- For those with very sensitive stomachs, the skin of the potato can be removed.
- Substitute chicken with any tolerated protein or additional vegetables as preferred.

Veggie Scramble

A colorful and nutritious start to the day, this veggie scramble is a light yet filling meal, packed with soft-cooked vegetables and eggs for easy digestion, perfect for those managing diabetic gastroparesis.

Preparation Time: 10 minutes
Cooking Time: 10 minutes
Servings: 1

Ingredients:
- 2 large eggs
- 1/4 cup diced bell peppers (well-cooked)
- 1/4 cup spinach, finely chopped and cooked
- 1 tablespoon olive oil
- Salt and pepper to taste

Directions:
1. Get your non-stick pan hot by heating up some olive oil over medium heat.
2. Add the well-cooked bell peppers and spinach to the skillet, sautéing for a minute until they are warmed through.
3. Beat the eggs with salt and pepper, then pour over the vegetables in the skillet.

4. Cook, stirring gently until the eggs are scrambled and fully cooked.
5. Serve immediately.

Nutritional Value Per Serving:
Calories: 250 | Carbs: 4g | Fiber: 1g | Protein: 14g | Sodium: 220mg | Sugar: 2g

Tips and Substitutions:
- You can substitute any tolerated vegetables.
- For a lower-fat option, use one whole egg and two egg whites instead of two whole eggs.

Cottage Cheese and Berries

This simple, no-cook recipe combines the creamy texture of cottage cheese with the natural sweetness of berries, providing a high-protein meal that's gentle on the stomach for those with diabetic gastroparesis.

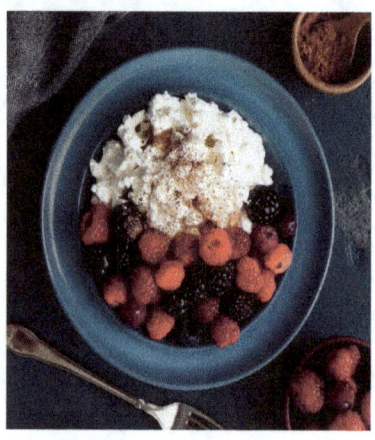

Preparation Time: 5 minutes
Cooking Time: 0 minutes
Servings: 1

Ingredients:
- 1/2 cup low-fat cottage cheese
- 1/2 cup berries (such as strawberries or blueberries, depending on tolerance)
- A drizzle of honey (optional)

Directions:
1. Place the cottage cheese in a serving bowl.

2. Top with the berries. Drizzle with honey if desired.
3. Serve immediately or chill in the refrigerator before serving.

Nutritional Value Per Serving:
Calories: 150 | Carbs: 15g | Fiber: 2g | Protein: 14g | Sodium: 350mg | Sugar: 10g

Tips and Substitutions:
- For those who need to avoid seeds, opt for seedless berry varieties or use tolerated fruit alternatives.
- You can also blend the cottage cheese for a smoother texture.

Cinnamon Apple Oatmeal

A comforting bowl of oatmeal enhanced with the warm flavors of cinnamon and apple, offering a fiber-rich yet easily digestible meal to start the day, ideal for managing diabetes and gastroparesis.

Preparation Time: 5 minutes
Cooking Time: 10 minutes
Servings: 1

Ingredients:
- 1/2 cup rolled oats
- 1 cup water or low-fat milk
- 1/2 apple, peeled and finely chopped
- 1/4 teaspoon cinnamon
- 1 teaspoon of honey or maple syrup (skip it if you want to keep it sugar-free!)

Directions:
1. In a small saucepan, heat the water or milk to a simmering boil. Add the oats and cinnamon, reducing the heat to a simmer.
2. Add the chopped apple to the pot. Cook, stirring occasionally, until the oats are soft and the mixture has thickened, about 5-10 minutes.

3. Remove from heat and let sit for a couple of minutes to cool slightly.
4. Stir in honey or maple syrup if using.
5. Serve warm.

Nutritional Value Per Serving:
Calories: 200 | Carbs: 38g | Fiber: 5g | Protein: 5g | Sodium: 50mg | Sugar: 12g

---

Tips and Substitutions:
- For a smoother texture, the apple can be cooked separately until very soft and then added to the oatmeal.
- Use any tolerated sweetener as an alternative to honey or maple syrup.

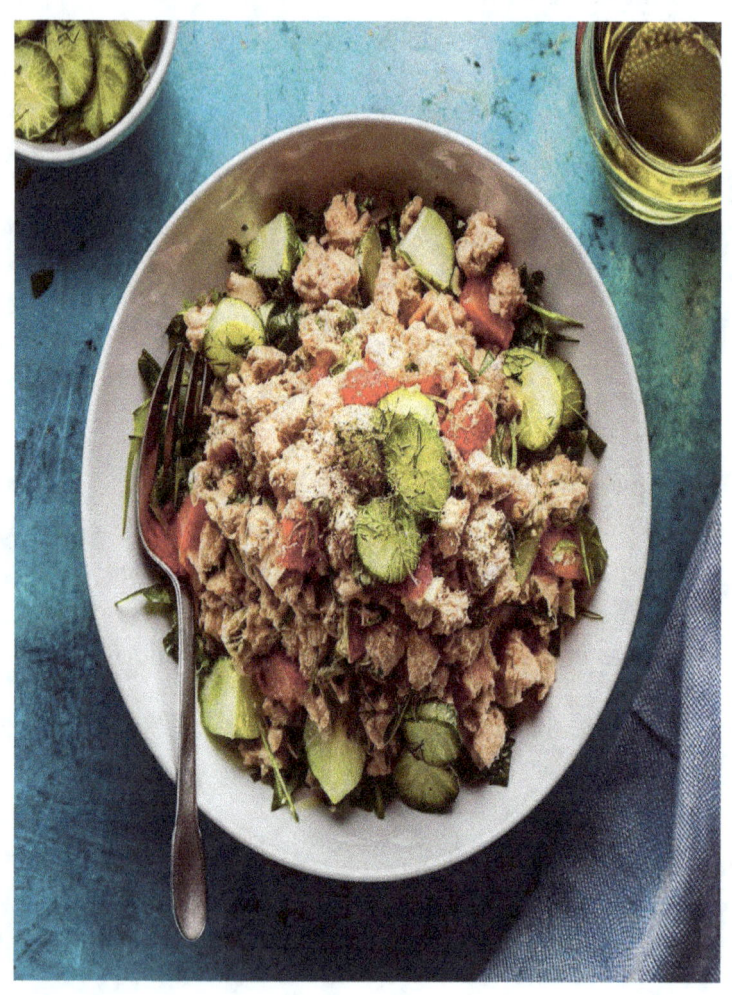

Chapter 5: Lunch Recipes

Vegetable Soup
Turkey Sandwich
Mushroom Chicken Marsala
Tuna Salad
Chia Pudding
Salmon with Roasted Asparagus
Egg Salad Lettuce Wraps
Chicken Caesar Lite
Hummus Veggie Wrap
Gazpacho

Vegetable Soup

A soothing and hydrating option for those with diabetic gastroparesis, this vegetable soup can be easily adjusted to include tolerated vegetables, offering both nutrition and comfort in every spoonful.

Preparation Time: 15 minutes
Cooking Time: 30 minutes
Servings: 4

Ingredients:
- 2 tablespoons olive oil
- 1/2 cup carrots, peeled and diced
- 1/2 cup zucchini, peeled and diced
- 1/2 cup spinach, finely chopped
- 4 cups low-sodium vegetable broth
- Salt and pepper to taste
- 1/2 teaspoon dried thyme

Directions:
1. On medium heat, warm the olive oil in a large pot. Add the carrots and cook for about 5 minutes, until slightly tender.
2. Add the zucchini and cook for another 5 minutes.

3. Pour in the vegetable broth, add the spinach, and season with thyme, salt, and pepper. Bring to a simmer.

4. Cook on low for 20 minutes, allowing the flavors to meld together.

5. Adjust seasoning as needed and serve hot.

Nutritional Value Per Serving:
Calories: 80 | Carbs: 10g | Fiber: 3g | Protein: 2g | Sodium: 150mg | Sugar: 4g

Tips and Substitutions:
- Any tolerated vegetables can be used.
- For a smoother soup, blend before serving.
- Add cooked, shredded chicken for extra protein if tolerated.

Turkey Sandwich

A simple and nutritious turkey sandwich on soft, whole-grain bread, packed with lean protein and easy-to-digest toppings, suitable for a diabetic gastroparesis diet.

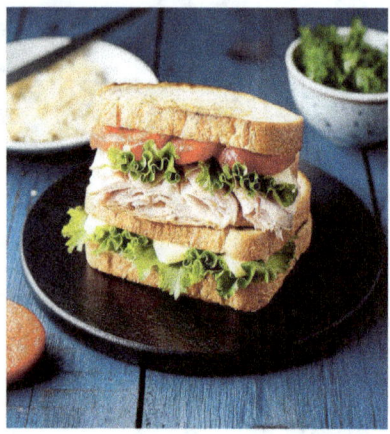

Preparation Time: 5 minutes
Cooking Time: 0 minutes
Servings: 1

Ingredients:
- 2 slices soft, whole-grain bread
- 3 ounces thinly sliced turkey breast
- 1 slice low-fat cheese
- Lettuce leaves (optional)
- Mustard or mayonnaise (optional)

Directions:
1. Lay the slices of bread on a clean surface.

2. Place the turkey slices on one piece of bread. Add the cheese and lettuce if using.
3. Spread a thin layer of mustard or mayonnaise on the other slice of bread, if desired.
4. Place the second slice of bread on top to form a sandwich.
5. Cut in half and serve.

Nutritional Value Per Serving:
Calories: 250 | Carbs: 20g | Fiber: 3g | Protein: 20g | Sodium: 700mg | Sugar: 5g

Tips and Substitutions:
- Use gluten-free bread if necessary.
- For a softer sandwich, remove the crusts or lightly toast the bread.
- Avoid raw vegetables if not tolerated; opt for avocado slices for added moisture and nutrition if tolerated.

Mushroom Chicken Marsala

Tender chicken breasts in a rich and savory Marsala wine sauce with mushrooms, this dish offers a sophisticated flavor profile while being mindful of the dietary needs of those with diabetic gastroparesis.

Preparation Time: 20 minutes
Cooking Time: 30 minutes
Servings: 4

Ingredients:
- 4 tenderized chicken breasts, without bones/skin
- Salt and pepper to taste
- 1/4 cup all-purpose flour (for dredging)
- 4 tablespoons unsalted butter
- 1 cup sliced mushrooms
- 3/4 cup Marsala wine
- 1/2 cup chicken broth
- Fresh parsley, chopped (for garnish)

Directions:
1. Sprinkle both sides of the chicken with salt and pepper. Then, coat the chicken evenly in flour.
2. Heat up 2 tablespoons of butter in a large skillet over medium heat. Once melted, add the chicken

breasts and cook until they're golden brown on both sides and cooked through. Then, take the chicken out of the pan and set it aside for a moment.

3. In the same skillet, add the remaining butter and mushrooms. Cook until the mushrooms are soft.

4. Add the Marsala wine and chicken broth, scraping up any browned bits from the pan. Let the sauce simmer undisturbed until it reduces in volume by about half.

5. Once the sauce is thickened, return the chicken breasts to the skillet and gently coat them in the flavorful sauce. . Heat through.

6. Garnish with parsley before serving.

Nutritional Value Per Serving:
Calories: 350 | Carbs: 12g | Fiber: 1g | Protein: 25g | Sodium: 200mg | Sugar: 2g

---

Tips and Substitutions:
- For a gluten-free option, use cornstarch instead of flour for dredging.
- Alcohol in the Marsala wine cooks off, but if preferred, use non-alcoholic wine or chicken broth with a bit of balsamic vinegar for a similar flavor profile.

Tuna Salad

A classic and versatile dish, this tuna salad combines flaked tuna with creamy mayonnaise and crisp, tolerated vegetables, perfect for a light lunch or snack for those on a diabetic gastroparesis diet.

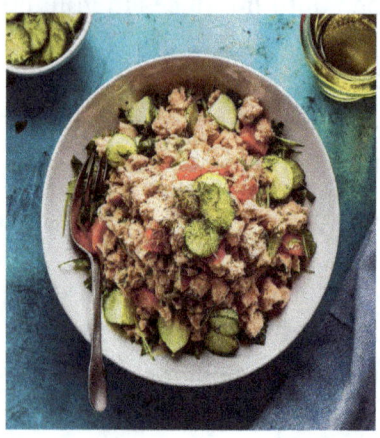

Preparation Time: 10 minutes
Cooking Time: 0 minutes
Servings: 2

Ingredients:
- 1 can (5 ounces) tuna in water, drained
- 2 tablespoons mayonnaise
- 1/4 cup finely diced celery (optional)
- Salt and pepper to taste
- Lettuce leaves or soft bread for serving

Directions:
1. In a bowl, mix the drained tuna, mayonnaise, and diced celery until well combined. Season with salt and pepper.

2. Serve the tuna salad on lettuce leaves for a low-carb option or spread between slices of soft bread for a sandwich.

Nutritional Value Per Serving:
Calories: 180 | Carbs: 1g | Fiber: 0g | Protein: 20g | Sodium: 390mg | Sugar: 1g

---

Tips and Substitutions:
- Swap out the mayo for Greek yogurt for a healthier twist.
- Omit celery if not tolerated and consider adding other tolerated vegetables or relish for crunch and flavor.

Chia Pudding

Chia pudding is a nutritious and easy-to-prepare option that's ideal for a gastroparesis-friendly diet. Rich in omega-3 fatty acids and fiber, it promotes heart health and digestion. Its smooth texture makes it easy to eat and digest.

Preparation Time: 5 minutes (plus at least 4 hours chilling)
Cooking Time: 0 minutes
Servings: 2

Ingredients:
- 1/4 cup chia seeds
- 1 cup almond milk or any non-dairy milk
- 1 tablespoon maple syrup or honey
- 1/2 teaspoon vanilla extract

Directions:
1. In a bowl, combine the chia seeds, almond milk, maple syrup, and vanilla extract.
2. Whisk until well combined.
3. Cover and refrigerate for at least 4 hours, or overnight, until it reaches a pudding-like consistency.

4. Stir once more before serving. Feel free to include more almond milk if needed for desired consistency.

Nutritional Value Per Serving:
Calories: 150 | Carbs: 15g | Fiber: 10g | Protein: 4g | Sodium: 95mg | Sugar: 5g

Tips and Substitutions:
- For a smoother texture, blend the pudding after it has set.
- Customize with tolerated toppings such as pureed fruits for additional flavor.

Salmon with Roasted Asparagus

This dish combines the rich flavors of salmon with the simplicity of roasted asparagus, providing a meal rich in omega-3 fatty acids, protein, and fiber, suitable for those managing both diabetes and gastroparesis.

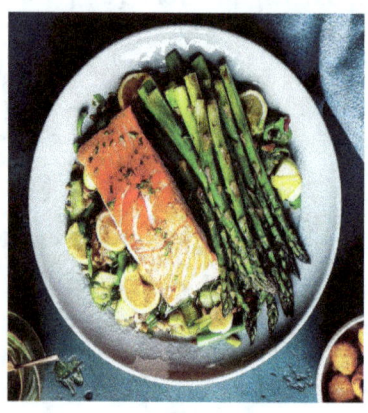

Preparation Time: 10 minutes
Cooking Time: 20 minutes
Servings: 2

Ingredients:
- 2 salmon fillets (about 6 ounces each)
- 1 tablespoon olive oil
- Salt and pepper to taste
- 1/2 pound asparagus, ends trimmed and peeled if thick

Directions:
1. Preheat the oven to 400°F (200°C).

2. Arrange the salmon and asparagus on a baking sheet. Add a drizzle of olive oil and sprinkle with salt and pepper to taste.
3. Roast for about 20 minutes, or until the salmon is cooked through and the asparagus is tender.
4. Serve immediately.

Nutritional Value Per Serving:
Calories: 345 | Carbs: 5g | Fiber: 2g | Protein: 34g | Sodium: 75mg | Sugar: 2g

---

Tips and Substitutions:
- For a softer vegetable option, asparagus can be steamed until very tender.
- Lemon zest or herbs like dill can be added for extra flavor without additional salt.

Egg Salad Lettuce Wraps

A fresh and light take on traditional egg salad, these lettuce wraps are perfect for a quick lunch. Packed with protein and nestled in crisp lettuce, they're a satisfying, easy-to-digest meal option for those with diabetic gastroparesis.

Preparation Time: 15 minutes
Cooking Time: 10 minutes
Servings: 2

Ingredients:
- 4 hard-boiled eggs, peeled and chopped
- 2 tablespoons mayonnaise
- Salt and pepper to taste
- Lettuce leaves, for serving

Directions:
1. In a bowl, combine the chopped eggs and mayonnaise. Season with salt and pepper to taste.
2. Mix until well combined.
3. Spoon the egg salad into lettuce leaves, folding them over to create wraps.
4. Serve immediately.

Nutritional Value Per Serving:
Calories: 230 | Carbs: 1g | Fiber: 0g |
Protein: 12g | Sodium: 310mg | Sugar: 1g

Tips and Substitutions:
- For a lower-fat version, use Greek yogurt instead of mayonnaise.
- Add herbs like dill or chives for extra flavor without increasing sodium content.

Chicken Caesar Lite

A lighter version of the classic Caesar salad, this recipe uses grilled chicken breast and a low-fat Caesar dressing over a bed of soft lettuce, making it suitable for those managing both diabetes and gastroparesis.

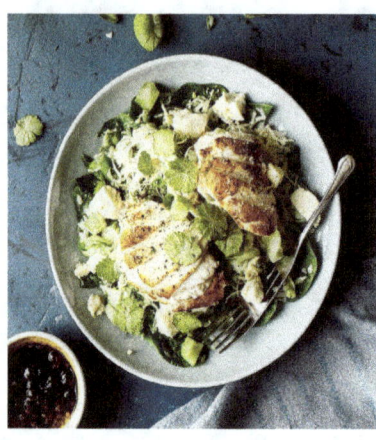

Preparation Time: 15 minutes
Cooking Time: 10 minutes
Servings: 2

Ingredients:
- 2 boneless, skinless chicken breasts
- Salt and pepper to taste
- 4 cups romaine lettuce, chopped (ensure it's tolerated)
- 1/4 cup low-fat Caesar dressing
- 2 tablespoons grated Parmesan cheese
- Lemon wedges for serving

Directions:
1. Season the chicken breasts with salt and pepper. Grill over medium heat for about 5 minutes on each side, until fully cooked. Let them rest for a couple of minutes before thinly slicing them.
2. In a large bowl, toss the chopped lettuce with Caesar dressing until well coated.
3. Divide the dressed lettuce between plates, top with sliced chicken, and sprinkle with Parmesan cheese.
4. Serve with lemon wedges on the side.

Nutritional Value Per Serving:
Calories: 300 | Carbs: 8g | Fiber: 2g | Protein: 38g | Sodium: 530mg | Sugar: 3g

---

Tips and Substitutions:
- For an even lighter version, substitute Caesar dressing with a mixture of lemon juice, olive oil, and a small amount of grated Parmesan.
- Avoid croutons to maintain a soft texture suitable for gastroparesis.

Hummus Veggie Wrap

This hummus veggie wrap offers a refreshing, no-cook meal option that's easy on the stomach and customizable based on individual tolerance levels. It combines the creaminess of hummus with the crunch of fresh vegetables, all wrapped in a soft tortilla for a light yet satisfying meal.

Preparation Time: 10 minutes
Cooking Time: 0 minutes
Servings: 2

Ingredients:
- 2 large soft tortillas (gluten-free if necessary)
- 4 tablespoons hummus
- 1/2 cucumber, thinly sliced (peeled if necessary)
- 1 carrot, grated (optional based on tolerance)
- 1/4 red bell pepper, thinly sliced (optional based on tolerance)
- A few leaves of soft lettuce

Directions:
1. Lay out the tortillas on a flat surface. Spread 2 tablespoons of hummus on each tortilla, leaving a small border around the edges.

2. Evenly distribute the cucumber, carrot, and red bell pepper slices over the hummus. Add a layer of soft lettuce.
3. Carefully roll up the tortillas, tucking in the sides as you go to keep the filling inside.
4. Cut the wraps in half and serve immediately.

Nutritional Value Per Serving:
Calories: 220 | Carbs: 35g | Fiber: 5g |
Protein: 8g | Sodium: 320mg | Sugar: 4g

Tips and Substitutions:
- Substitute any of the vegetables with other tolerated options, such as spinach or roasted vegetables for a different flavor profile.
- For a gluten-free option, ensure the tortillas are made from gluten-free grains.

Gazpacho

Gazpacho is a chilled, blended soup traditionally made from ripe tomatoes and a variety of vegetables. For individuals with diabetic gastroparesis, this recipe is adjusted to reduce fiber and ensure it's well-puréed to ease digestion, offering a nutritious, hydrating, and refreshing meal or side dish.

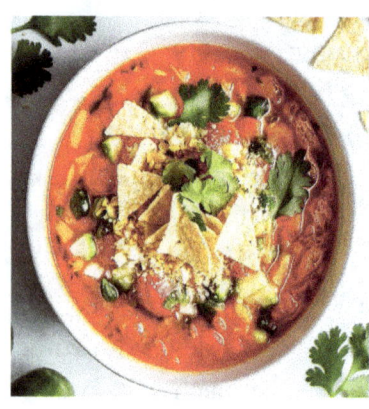

Preparation Time: 15 minutes (plus chilling)
Cooking Time: 0 minutes
Servings: 4

Ingredients:
- 4 juicy ripe tomatoes, with the skin and seeds removed
- 1/2 cucumber, peeled and seeded
- 1/2 red bell pepper, cored and seeded
- 1 small garlic clove, minced (optional, based on tolerance)
- 2 tablespoons extra virgin olive oil
- 1 tablespoon red wine vinegar
- Salt and pepper to taste
- 1 cup cold water

Directions:

1. In a blender, combine the tomatoes, cucumber, red bell pepper, garlic (if using), olive oil, red wine vinegar, and a pinch of salt and pepper. Blend until smooth.
2. While blending, gradually add up to 1 cup of cold water until you reach your desired consistency.
3. Taste and adjust seasoning as necessary.
4. Chill in the refrigerator for at least 2 hours before serving.
5. Serve cold, garnished with diced cucumber or a drizzle of olive oil, if desired.

Nutritional Value Per Serving:
Calories: 100 | Carbs: 8g | Fiber: 2g | Protein: 2g | Sodium: 20mg | Sugar: 6g

Tips and Substitutions:

- For an even smoother texture, pass the blended soup through a sieve.
- Adjust the amount of garlic or omit it altogether to suit tolerance.
- For extra flavor, add a small amount of low-sodium vegetable broth in place of some of the water.

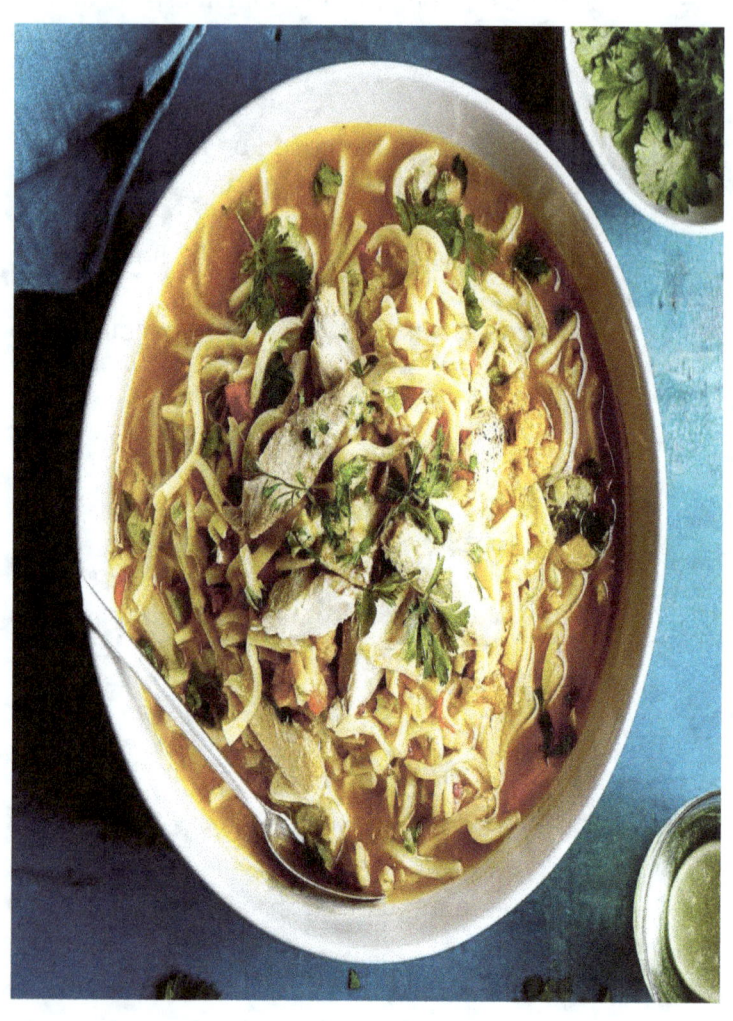

Chapter 6: Dinner Recipes

Cauliflower Soup
Baked Fish with Lemon and Herbs
Chicken and Vegetable Stir-Fry
Egg Salad with Whole Grain Crackers
Baked Sweet Potato with Cinnamon and Butter
Quinoa Salad with Roasted Vegetables
Spaghetti Squash with Marinara Sauce
Delicious Simple Soup
Zucchini Bake
Chicken Noodle

Cauliflower Soup

Cauliflower soup is a creamy, comforting dish perfect for those with diabetic gastroparesis, offering a smooth texture that's easy on the stomach. It's low in carbs and can be enriched with protein if desired.

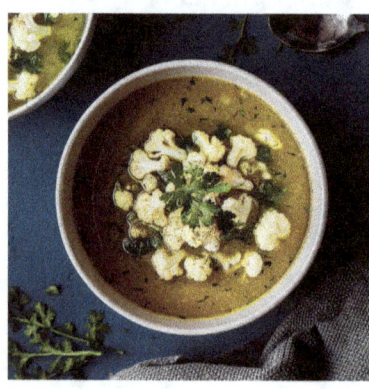

Preparation Time: 10 minutes
Cooking Time: 20 minutes
Servings: 4

Ingredients:
- 1 medium head cauliflower, chopped
- 1 tablespoon olive oil
- 1 small onion, finely chopped (optional, based on tolerance)
- 2 cloves garlic, minced (optional, based on tolerance)
- 3 cups of chicken or vegetable broth, (low-sodium version)
- 1/2 cup light cream or milk alternative
- Salt and pepper to taste

Directions:
1. Warm the olive oil in a large pot over medium heat. Add the onion and garlic (if using) and sauté until soft and translucent.
2. Add the cauliflower and broth. Bring to a boil, then reduce the heat and simmer until the cauliflower is very tender, about 15 minutes.
3. Use your immersion blender to achieve a creamy consistency for the soup. Stir in the light cream, and season with salt and pepper to taste.
4. Heat through, then serve warm.

Nutritional Value Per Serving:
Calories: 110 | Carbs: 10g | Fiber: 3g |
Protein: 5g | Sodium: 150mg | Sugar: 4g

Tips and Substitutions:
- To keep it dairy-free, swap in almond milk or coconut milk.
- If onions and garlic are not tolerated, enhance flavor with a pinch of nutmeg or herbs like thyme.

Baked Fish with Lemon and Herbs

This baked fish recipe is simple, flavorful, and gentle on the stomach, making it ideal for those managing diabetic gastroparesis. Using lean fish and fresh herbs, it offers a high-quality protein source with minimal fat.

Preparation Time: 5 minutes
Cooking Time: 12-15 minutes
Servings: 2

Ingredients:
- 2 fish fillets (e.g., tilapia, cod)
- 2 tablespoons olive oil
- 1 lemon, sliced
- Fresh herbs (e.g., dill, parsley), chopped
- Salt and pepper to taste

Directions:
1. Preheat the oven to 400°F (200°C). Prep your baking sheet by laying down a sheet of parchment paper.
2. Place the fish fillets on the prepared baking sheet. Lightly coat with olive oil and sprinkle with salt and pepper.

3. Top each fillet with lemon slices and chopped herbs.
4. Bake in the preheated oven for 12-15 minutes, or until the fish flakes easily with a fork.
5. Serve immediately, garnished with additional herbs if desired.

Nutritional Value Per Serving:
Calories: 220 | Carbs: 1g | Fiber: 0g | Protein: 25g | Sodium: 70mg | Sugar: 0g

Tips and Substitutions:
- To avoid citrus, use a small amount of vinegar for acidity.
- If fresh herbs aren't available, dried herbs can be a good substitute; use them sparingly to avoid overpowering the fish.

Chicken and Vegetable Stir-Fry

A quick and easy meal that's customizable to your dietary needs, this chicken and vegetable stir-fry provides a satisfying mix of lean protein and soft-cooked vegetables, seasoned with gentle flavors.

Preparation Time: 10 minutes
Cooking Time: 10 minutes
Servings: 2

Ingredients:
- 2 chicken breasts, thinly sliced
- 2 cups mixed vegetables (e.g., carrots, zucchini), cut into small pieces
- 1 tablespoon olive oil
- 2 tablespoons low-sodium soy sauce
- Salt and pepper to taste
- Cooked/steamed rice or noodles, for serving (optional)

Directions:
1. Heat the olive oil in a large pan or wok over medium-high heat.
2. Add the chicken slices and stir-fry until they start to brown.

3. Add the vegetables and continue to stir-fry until the vegetables are tender but still crisp.
4. Pour in the soy sauce, and season with salt and pepper. Stir well to combine.
5. Serve hot over rice or noodles if tolerated.

Nutritional Value Per Serving:
Calories: 300 | Carbs: 8g | Fiber: 2g |
Protein: 36g | Sodium: 620mg | Sugar: 4g

Tips and Substitutions:
- For a soy-free option, use coconut aminos instead of soy sauce.
- Ensure vegetables are cooked until very tender to make them easier to digest.
- Choose vegetables that are tolerated well.

Egg Salad with Whole Grain Crackers

Egg salad paired with whole-grain crackers offers a nutrient-rich meal or snack, providing both protein and complex carbohydrates. This combination can be tailored to individual tolerance levels, making it a versatile option for those with diabetic gastroparesis.

Preparation Time: 10 minutes
Cooking Time: 10 minutes (for the eggs)
Servings: 2

Ingredients:
- 4 hard-boiled eggs, peeled and chopped
- 2 tablespoons mayonnaise
- Salt and pepper to taste
- Whole grain crackers for serving

Directions:
1. In a bowl, combine the chopped eggs with mayonnaise. Mash together with a fork. Season with salt and pepper to taste.
2. Serve the egg salad with whole grain crackers on the side.

Nutritional Value Per Serving:
Calories: 280 | Carbs: 12g | Fiber: 2g |
Protein: 14g | Sodium: 320mg | Sugar: 2g

Tips and Substitutions:
- For a lighter version, use Greek yogurt instead of mayonnaise.
- If whole grain crackers are not tolerated, serve with soft bread or by itself.
- Add herbs like dill or chives for extra flavor without adding bulk.

Baked Sweet Potato with Cinnamon and Butter

A baked sweet potato with cinnamon and butter is a comforting, nutritious dish perfect for those with diabetic gastroparesis. It provides a good source of vitamins, fiber, and flavor, with a soft texture that is generally well tolerated.

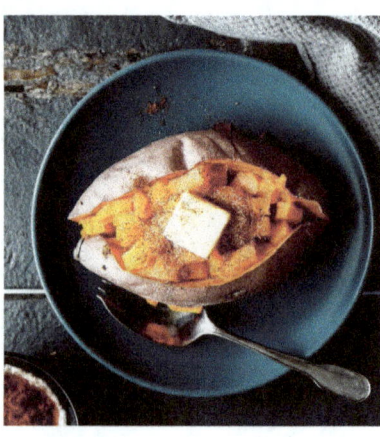

Preparation Time: 5 minutes
Cooking Time: 45 minutes
Servings: 2

Ingredients:
- 2 medium sweet potatoes, scrubbed
- 2 teaspoons butter
- 1/2 teaspoon ground cinnamon
- Salt to taste

Directions:
1. Preheat the oven to 400°F (200°C).

2. Prick the sweet potatoes several times with a fork and place them on a baking sheet.
3. Bake in the preheated oven until tender, about 45 minutes.
4. Split the tops of the sweet potatoes with a knife. Fluff the insides with a fork.
5. Top each sweet potato with 1 teaspoon of butter, a sprinkle of cinnamon, and a pinch of salt.
6. Serve warm.

Nutritional Value Per Serving:
Calories: 160 | Carbs: 26g | Fiber: 4g | Protein: 2g | Sodium: 150mg | Sugar: 5g

Tips and Substitutions:
- To create a vegan option, substitute with a dairy-free spread.
- To add more protein, top with a dollop of Greek yogurt.

Quinoa Salad with Roasted Vegetables

This quinoa salad with roasted vegetables is a nutritious, fiber-rich dish that's easy to customize for those with diabetic gastroparesis. Quinoa provides a complete protein source, while the vegetables add vitamins and minerals.

Preparation Time: 15 minutes
Cooking Time: 25 minutes
Servings: 4

Ingredients:
- 1 cup quinoa, rinsed
- 2 cups water
- 2 cups mixed vegetables (e.g., bell peppers, zucchini), diced
- 1 tablespoon olive oil
- 1 teaspoon dried herbs (e.g., thyme, oregano)
- Salt and pepper to taste
- 2 tablespoons lemon juice

Directions:
1. Preheat the oven to 400°F (200°C). Toss the diced vegetables with olive oil, herbs, salt, and

pepper. Spread on a baking sheet and roast until tender, about 25 minutes.
2. Meanwhile, combine quinoa and water in a pot. Bring to a boil, then cover, reduce heat to low, and simmer for 15 minutes, or until the water is absorbed. Take off the heat and let it stand covered for 5 minutes.
3. Fluff the quinoa with a fork and transfer to a large bowl. Add the roasted vegetables and lemon juice. Toss to combine.
4. Season with additional salt and pepper if needed and serve warm or at room temperature.

Nutritional Value Per Serving:
Calories: 220 | Carbs: 38g | Fiber: 5g | Protein: 8g | Sodium: 30mg | Sugar: 3g

---

Tips and Substitutions:
- For easier digestion, ensure the vegetables are well-roasted and soft.
- Substitute any of the vegetables with others that are better tolerated.
- Add a handful of chopped fresh herbs before serving for extra flavor.

Spaghetti Squash with Marinara Sauce

Spaghetti squash with marinara sauce is a light, diabetes-friendly alternative to traditional pasta dishes. It offers the comfort of spaghetti without the heavy carbs, making it suitable for those with diabetic gastroparesis.

Preparation Time: 10 minutes
Cooking Time: 40 minutes
Servings: 4

Ingredients:
- 1 medium spaghetti squash
- 1 tablespoon olive oil
- 2 cups marinara sauce (low-sodium, no added sugar)
- Salt and pepper to taste
- Grated Parmesan cheese (optional)

Directions:
1. Preheat the oven to 400°F (200°C). Halve the spaghetti squash lengthwise and remove the seeds.
2. Brush the cut surfaces with olive oil and sprinkle with salt and pepper. Then, lay the squash halves face-down on a baking sheet.

3. Bake until the flesh is tender and easily shreds with a fork, about 40 minutes.
4. Remove from the oven, let cool slightly, then use a fork to scrape the squash into strands.
5. Heat the marinara sauce in a saucepan over medium heat until warm.
6. Serve the spaghetti squash topped with marinara sauce and grated Parmesan cheese, if using.

**Nutritional Value Per Serving:
Calories: 140 | Carbs: 20g | Fiber: 4g |
Protein: 3g | Sodium: 320mg | Sugar: 8g**

Tips and Substitutions:
- For added protein, mix in cooked ground turkey or tofu into the marinara sauce.
- Choose a marinara sauce with no added sugars and low sodium to keep it diabetes-friendly.

Delicious Simple Soup

This delicious simple soup is designed to be gentle on the stomach while providing hydration and nutrients. It's versatile and can be adapted to include tolerated vegetables and protein sources.

Preparation Time: 10 minutes
Cooking Time: 20 minutes
Servings: 4

Ingredients:
- 4 cups vegetable or chicken broth (low-sodium version)
- 1 cup mixed vegetables (carrots, zucchini), diced
- 1 cup cooked protein (chicken, tofu, lentils, etc.), diced or shredded (optional)
- 1/2 cup cooked quinoa or rice (optional)
- Salt and pepper to taste
- Fresh herbs (e.g., parsley, dill) for garnish

Directions:
1. In a large pot, bring the vegetable or chicken broth to a simmer over medium heat.

2. Add the diced mixed vegetables and cooked protein, if using. Let the vegetables simmer for 10-15 minutes, or until they become tender.
3. If adding cooked quinoa or rice, stir it into the soup and cook for an additional 5 minutes.
4. Adjust the soup's flavor with salt and pepper as desired.
5. Ladle the soup into bowls, garnish with fresh herbs, and serve hot.

Nutritional Value Per Serving (Without Optional Ingredients):
Calories: 40 | Carbs: 8g | Fiber: 2g | Protein: 1g | Sodium: 100mg | Sugar: 2g

---

Tips and Substitutions:
- Customize the soup with tolerated vegetables and protein sources.
- For a thicker soup, blend a portion of it and mix it back into the pot.
- Add a squeeze of lemon juice for extra flavor without added sodium.
- Use fresh or dried herbs for garnishing based on preference and availability.

Zucchini Bake

Zucchini bake is a light and flavorful dish that's gentle on the stomach and suitable for those with diabetic gastroparesis. It combines zucchini with a savory filling, baked to perfection for a satisfying meal.

Preparation Time: 15 minutes
Cooking Time: 35 minutes
Servings: 4

Ingredients:
- 2 large zucchinis, sliced lengthwise
- 1 cup cooked quinoa or rice
- 1/2 cup grated Parmesan cheese
- 1/2 cup marinara sauce (low-sodium, no added sugar)
- 1/4 cup chopped fresh basil
- Salt and pepper to taste
- Olive oil for greasing

Directions:
1. Preheat the oven to 375°F (190°C). Lightly coat a baking dish with olive oil.
2. Arrange the zucchini slices in the bottom of the baking dish.

3. In a bowl, combine the cooked quinoa or rice, grated Parmesan cheese, marinara sauce, chopped basil, salt, and pepper. Mix well.
4. Spread the quinoa or rice mixture evenly over the zucchini slices.
5. Cover the baking dish with foil and bake for 25 minutes.
6. Remove the foil and bake for an additional 10 minutes, or until the top is golden brown and bubbly.
7. Serve hot, garnished with extra basil if desired.

Nutritional Value Per Serving:
Calories: 180 | Carbs: 18g | Fiber: 3g | Protein: 8g | Sodium: 250mg | Sugar: 4g

---

Tips and Substitutions:
- Customize the filling with tolerated ingredients such as cooked chicken or tofu for added protein.
- Use low-sodium marinara sauce to control sodium levels.
- For a hint of savory, cheesy taste without dairy, add a dusting of nutritional yeast.

Chicken Noodle

Chicken noodle soup is a classic comfort dish, and this version is modified to be easy on the stomach and suitable for those with diabetic gastroparesis. It combines tender chicken, soft noodles, and gentle flavors in a soothing broth.

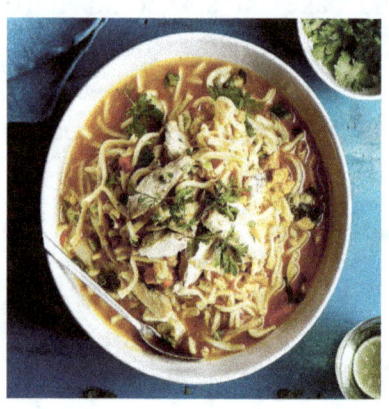

Preparation Time: 15 minutes
Cooking Time: 25 minutes
Servings: 4

Ingredients:
- 2 boneless, skinless chicken breasts, diced
- 6 cups low-sodium chicken broth
- 1 cup cooked noodles (e.g., egg noodles, rice noodles)
- 1 cup mixed vegetables (carrots, celery), diced
- 1/2 onion, chopped (optional, based on tolerance)
- 2 cloves garlic, minced (optional, based on tolerance)
- Salt and pepper to taste
- Fresh parsley for garnish

Directions:
1. Heat the chicken broth in a large pot over medium heat until it simmers gently.
2. Add the diced chicken, cooked noodles, mixed vegetables, onion (if using), and garlic (if using). Simmer until the chicken is cooked through and the vegetables are tender, about 20 minutes.
3. Adjust the soup's flavor with salt and pepper as desired.
4. Ladle the soup into bowls, garnish with fresh parsley, and serve hot.

Nutritional Value Per Serving:
Calories: 220 | Carbs: 15g | Fiber: 2g |
Protein: 25g | Sodium: 250mg | Sugar: 3g

Tips and Substitutions:
- Opt for low-sodium chicken broth to keep the sodium level in check.
- Choose soft noodles that are easily digestible, such as rice noodles or egg noodles.
- Customize the soup with additional tolerated vegetables or herbs for added flavor.

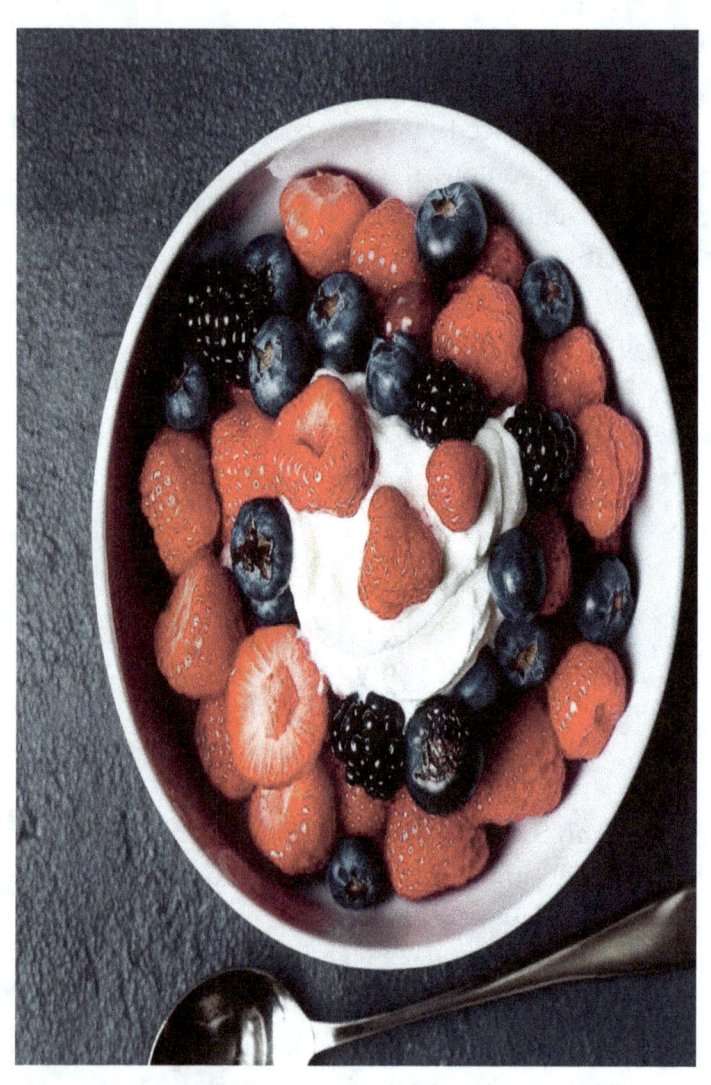

Chapter 7: Dessert/Snack Recipes

Almond and Date Energy Balls
Celery and Peanut Butter
Greek Yogurt with Berries and Chia Seeds
Greek Yogurt Parfait
Berries and Cream
Cucumber and Hummus
Baked Apples
Cottage Cheese Fruit Bowl
Trail Mix
Banana Ice Cream

Almond and Date Energy Balls

These energy balls are a nutritious, gastroparesis-friendly snack. Made with almonds and dates, they provide a natural energy boost without spiking blood sugar levels.

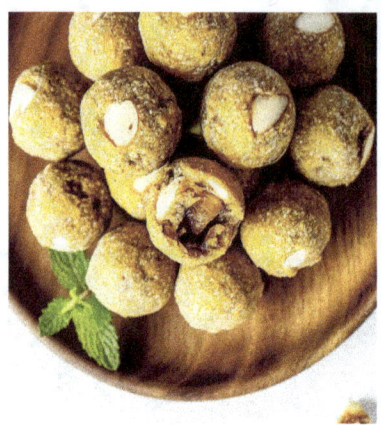

Preparation Time: 15 minutes
Cooking Time: 0 minutes
Servings: 8

Ingredients:
- 1 cup almonds
- 1 cup dates, pitted
- 1/4 cup shredded coconut (unsweetened)
- 1 tablespoon chia seeds
- 1 teaspoon vanilla extract

Directions:
1. In a food processor, blend almonds until finely chopped.

2. Add dates, shredded coconut, chia seeds, and vanilla extract. Process until the mixture sticks together.

3. Scoop out the mixture and roll into balls, about 1 inch in diameter.

4. Let it chill in the refrigerator for at least 1 hour before serving.

Nutritional Value Per Serving:
Calories: 150 | Carbs: 18g | Fiber: 3g | Protein: 4g | Sodium: 5mg | Sugar: 14g

Tips and Substitutions:
- Substitute almonds with any other nuts or seeds tolerated.
- Add a pinch of cinnamon or cocoa powder for variety.

Celery and Peanut Butter

A classic, simple snack that pairs the crunchiness of celery with the creamy richness of peanut butter. It's suitable for a gastroparesis diet and offers a good balance of fat and protein.

Prep Time: 5 minutes | Cooking Time: 0 minutes | Servings: 1

Ingredients:
- 2 celery stalks
- 2 tablespoons peanut butter (smooth or crunchy)

Directions:
1. Wash and dry the celery stalks.
2. Spread peanut butter evenly inside the celery groove.
3. Serve immediately.

Nutritional Value Per Serving:
Calories: 190 | Carbs: 8g | Fiber: 3g | Protein: 8g | Sodium: 150mg | Sugar: 4g

---

Tips and Substitutions:
- Use almond butter or sunflower seed butter as an alternative to peanut butter.

Greek Yogurt with Berries and Chia Seeds

Greek yogurt with berries and chia seeds is a nutritious and filling snack or breakfast option. It combines the creaminess of Greek yogurt with the sweetness of fresh berries and the added nutritional boost of chia seeds.

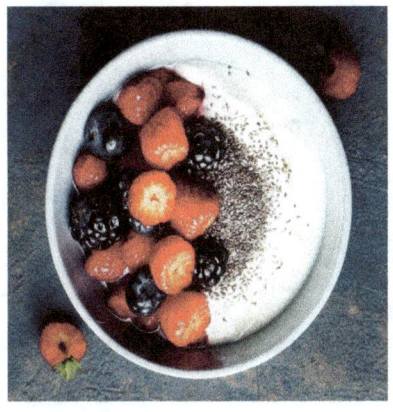

Preparation Time: 5 minutes
Cooking Time: 0 minutes
Servings: 1

Ingredients:
- 1/2 cup Greek yogurt (plain, low-fat or regular)
- 1/2 cup mixed berries (like strawberries, blueberries, raspberries)
- 1 tablespoon chia seeds
- 1 tablespoon honey or maple syrup (add this if you prefer a sweeter taste)

Directions:
1. In a serving bowl, place Greek yogurt.
2. Top with mixed berries.
3. Sprinkle chia seeds evenly over the berries.
4. Drizzle honey or maple syrup on top for added sweetness if desired.
5. Serve immediately.

Nutritional Value Per Serving:
Calories: 200 | Carbs: 24g | Fiber: 6g | Protein: 15g | Sodium: 55mg | Sugar: 16g

Tips and Substitutions:
- Use flavored Greek yogurt for added variety.
- Substitute chia seeds with ground flaxseeds if preferred.
- For an additional flavor boost, you can add a touch of cinnamon or nutmeg.

Greek Yogurt Parfait

A delightful and nutritious parfait that layers Greek yogurt with fruits and granola, providing a perfect balance of protein, fiber, and vitamins.

Preparation Time: 10 minutes
Cooking Time: 0 minutes
Servings: 1

Ingredients:
- 3/4 cup Greek yogurt (plain, low-fat)
- 1/2 cup mixed berries (think strawberries, blueberries, raspberries)
- 1/4 cup granola (low-fat, low-sugar)
- 1 tablespoon honey (optional)

Directions:
1. In a glass or bowl, layer half of the Greek yogurt.
2. Add a layer of mixed berries.
3. Scatter half the granola on top of the berries.
4. Repeat the layers with the remaining yogurt, berries, and granola.
5. Drizzle with honey if desired and serve immediately.

Nutritional Value Per Serving:
**Calories: 280 | Carbs: 36g | Fiber: 4g |
Protein: 20g | Sodium: 70mg | Sugar: 25g**

Tips and Substitutions:
- Choose low-fat, plain Greek yogurt to minimize fat content.
- For a smoother texture, blend the berries into a puree before layering.
- Substitute granola with tolerated nuts or seeds for a crunchy texture.

Berries and Cream

Berries and cream is a simple yet delicious dessert or snack that combines the sweetness of fresh berries with a creamy topping, perfect for those with gastroparesis.

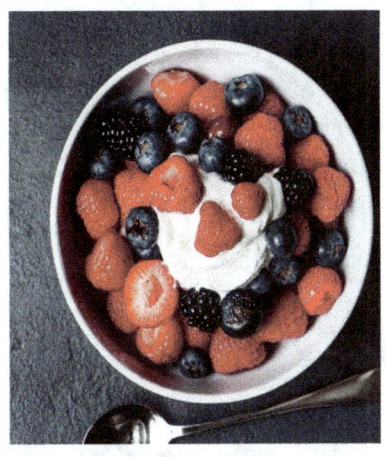

Preparation Time: 5 minutes
Cooking Time: 0 minutes
Servings: 1

Ingredients:
- 1/2 cup mixed berries such as strawberries, blueberries, raspberries
- 1/4 cup whipped cream or whipped coconut cream
- 1 teaspoon honey or maple syrup (optional)

Directions:
1. Wash and dry the berries.
2. Place the mixed berries in a bowl or serving dish.

3. Top with whipped cream or whipped coconut cream.
4. Drizzle with honey or maple syrup if desired.
5. Serve immediately.

Nutritional Value Per Serving:
Calories: 100 | Carbs: 10g | Fiber: 3g | Protein: 1g | Sodium: 10mg | Sugar: 7g

Tips and Substitutions:
- Feel free to use fresh or frozen berries, depending on what's easiest to find.
- For a dairy-free option, use whipped coconut cream.

Cucumber and Hummus

Cucumber and hummus make a refreshing and nutritious snack that's easy on the stomach. It combines hydrating cucumber with protein-rich hummus for a satisfying treat.

Prep Time: 5 minutes | Cooking Time: 0 minutes | Servings: 1

Ingredients:
- 1 medium cucumber, sliced
- 1/4 cup hummus (store-bought or homemade)

Directions:
1. Wash and slice the cucumber into rounds or sticks.
2. Serve the cucumber slices with a side of hummus for dipping.

Nutritional Value Per Serving:
Calories: 120 | Carbs: 12g | Fiber: 3g | Protein: 5g | Sodium: 150mg | Sugar: 2g

---

Tips and Substitutions:
- Use flavored hummus for added variety.
- Add a sprinkle of paprika or black pepper on the hummus for extra flavor.

Baked Apples

Baked apples are a warm and comforting dessert option that's gentle on the stomach. They can be flavored with cinnamon and served with a dollop of yogurt or a sprinkle of nuts.

Preparation Time: 10 minutes
Cooking Time: 30 minutes
Servings: 2

Ingredients:
- 2 medium apples, such as Granny Smith (tart) or Honeycrisp (sweet)
- 1 tablespoon butter or coconut oil
- 1 teaspoon ground cinnamon
- 1 tablespoon honey or maple syrup (optional)
- 2 tablespoons chopped nuts (walnuts, almonds) (optional)
- Greek yogurt or whipped coconut cream for serving (optional)

Directions:
1. Preheat the oven to 375°F (190°C).
2. Core the apples and place them in a baking dish.
3. In a small bowl, mix the melted butter or coconut oil with cinnamon and honey or maple syrup.

4. Pour the mixture over the apples, ensuring they are coated evenly.

5. Bake for 25-30 minutes, or until the apples are tender.

6. Take it out of the oven and let it rest for a few minutes to cool down a bit.

7. Serve warm, topped with chopped nuts and a dollop of Greek yogurt or whipped coconut cream if desired.

Nutritional Value Per Serving:
Calories: 180 | Carbs: 30g | Fiber: 5g | Protein: 2g | Sodium: 10mg | Sugar: 22g

---

Tips and Substitutions:

- Adjust the sweetness by using less honey or maple syrup.
- For an extra touch of crunchiness, top with a sprinkle of granola.

Cottage Cheese Fruit Bowl

A cottage cheese fruit bowl is a protein-rich and satisfying snack or breakfast option. It combines creamy cottage cheese with fresh fruits for a balanced and nutritious meal.

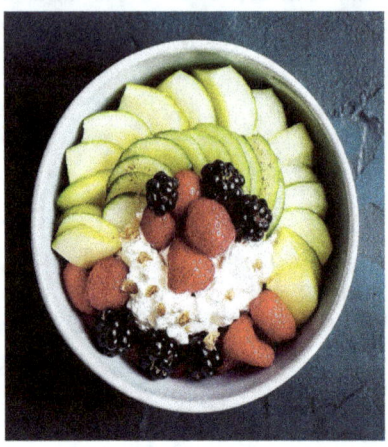

Preparation Time: 5 minutes
Cooking Time: 0 minutes
Servings: 1

Ingredients:
- 1/2 cup cottage cheese (low-fat or regular)
- 1/2 cup mixed fruits (such as berries, banana slices, or diced apples)
- 1 tablespoon honey or maple syrup (if you prefer the sweeter version)
- 1 tablespoon chopped nuts (optional)

Directions:
1. Place the cottage cheese in a bowl.

2. Top with mixed fruits.
3. Drizzle with honey or maple syrup if desired.
4. Sprinkle chopped nuts on top for added texture and flavor.

Nutritional Value Per Serving:
Calories: 180 | Carbs: 20g | Fiber: 3g | Protein: 15g | Sodium: 350mg | Sugar: 15g

---

Tips and Substitutions:
- Use Greek yogurt as a substitute for cottage cheese if preferred.
- Add a dash of cinnamon for extra flavor.
- Experiment with different fruit combinations based on availability and taste preferences.

Trail Mix

Trail mix is a versatile and customizable snack perfect for energy boosts. It combines nuts, seeds, and dried fruits for a portable and gastroparesis-friendly option.

Preparation Time: 5 minutes
Cooking Time: 0 minutes
Servings: 4

Ingredients:
- 1/2 cup almonds, lightly toasted
- 1/2 cup lightly toasted pecans or walnuts
- 1/4 cup pumpkin seeds
- 1/4 cup sunflower seeds
- 1/2 cup dried cranberries or raisins
- 1/4 cup mini dark chocolate chips (highly optional)

Directions:
1. In a large bowl, mix together almonds, walnuts or pecans, pumpkin seeds, sunflower seeds, and dried cranberries or raisins.
2. If using, stir in the mini dark chocolate chips.
3. Divide the mix into individual servings or store in an airtight container.

Nutritional Value Per Serving:
Calories: 300 | Carbs: 20g | Fiber: 4g | Protein: 7g | Sodium: 5mg | Sugar: 12g

Tips and Substitutions:
- Roast nuts and seeds at 350°F (175°C) for 10 minutes for extra flavor.
- Swap in any preferred nuts, seeds, or dried fruits.
- For a lower sugar option, omit the chocolate chips or use cacao nibs.

Banana Ice Cream

Banana ice cream, or "nice cream," is a simple, healthy dessert made from frozen bananas. It's a great alternative to traditional ice cream, offering natural sweetness and a creamy texture without added sugars or fats.

Preparation Time: 5 minutes (plus freezing time)
Cooking Time: 0 minutes
Servings: 2

Ingredients:
- 2 large ripe bananas, sliced and frozen
- 2-3 tablespoons almond milk or milk of choice (adjust for desired consistency)
- Optional add-ins: 1 tablespoon peanut butter, a dash of vanilla extract, or 1 tablespoon cocoa powder

Directions:
1. Pop those frozen banana slices into your food processor or a powerful blender.
2. Add a little almond milk and any optional add-ins.

3. Blend until smooth, creamy, and resembles soft serve ice cream. Gradually add more milk until it reaches your desired texture.

4. Serve immediately for a soft serve texture, or transfer to a freezer-safe container and freeze until solid for a firmer texture.

Nutritional Value Per Serving:
Calories: 105 | Carbs: 27g | Fiber: 3g |
Protein: 1g | Sodium: 1mg | Sugar: 14g

Tips and Substitutions:
- Freeze the bananas for at least 4 hours or overnight for the best texture.
- Experiment with mix-ins like fresh berries, chocolate chips, or nuts after blending for added flavor and texture.
- For a chocolate version, blend in 1 tablespoon of cocoa powder.

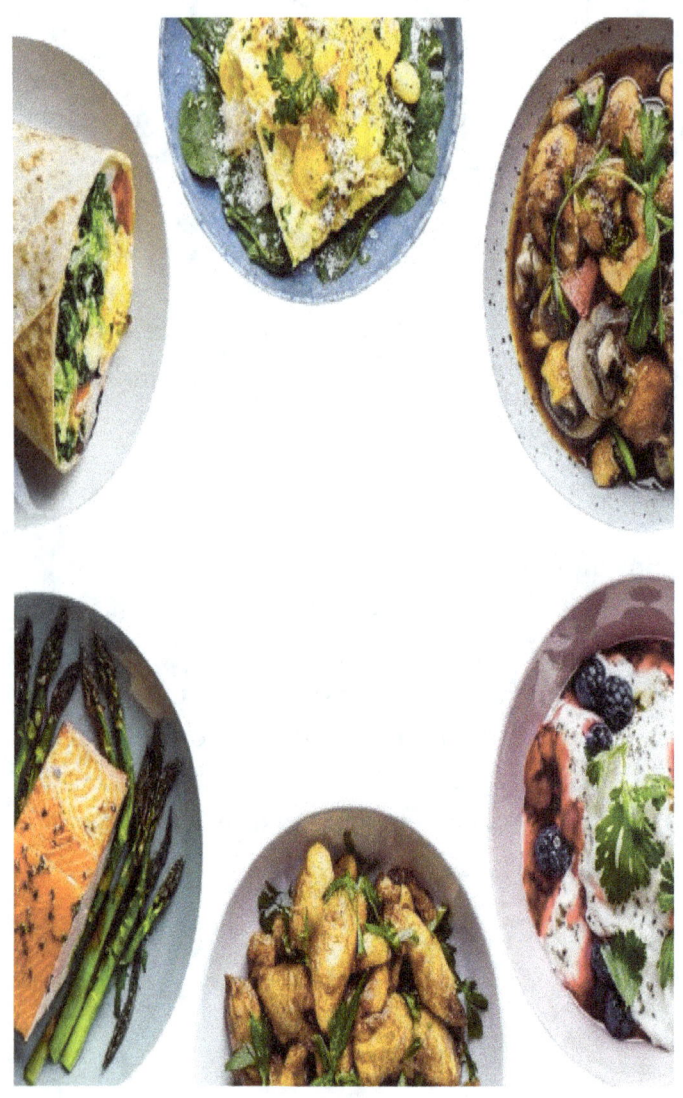

Chapter 8: Living Well with Diabetic Gastroparesis

Diabetic gastroparesis (DGP) can be a frustrating condition, but it doesn't have to define your life. This chapter explores strategies beyond diet that can help you manage DGP symptoms and maintain a positive outlook.

Tips for Managing Nausea and Vomiting

Nausea and vomiting are common symptoms of DGP, but there are ways to manage them:

- **Ginger**: Ginger is a natural remedy known to soothe nausea. Try ginger tea, sucking on ginger candies, or adding a sprinkle of ginger powder to your meals.
- **Acupressure**: Acupressure is like a massage, but instead of rubbing your whole body, you press on certain spots to help you feel better. A technique called P6 acupressure, which involves applying pressure to a point on your inner wrist, may help relieve nausea.

- **Relaxation Techniques**: Stress can worsen nausea. Consider relaxation techniques like deep breathing exercises or meditation to manage stress and potentially reduce your symptoms.
- **Medication**: Your doctor might prescribe medications to help control nausea and vomiting.

Maintaining a Positive Attitude

Living with a chronic condition like DGP can be challenging, but maintaining a positive attitude can significantly impact your well-being. Here are some tips:

- **Focus on What You Can Control**: You may not be able to control DGP itself, but you can control your diet, exercise routine, and stress management strategies. Instead of dwelling on problems, target the areas you can improve!
- **Connect with Others**: Talking to others who understand what you're going through can be incredibly helpful. Consider joining a support group for people with diabetes or DGP.
- **Celebrate Small Victories**: Managing DGP is a journey with ups and downs. Celebrate

even small victories, like a day with minimal nausea or successfully trying a new recipe.
- **Seek Professional Help**: If you're struggling to cope emotionally with DGP, don't hesitate to seek professional help from a therapist or counselor.

Cooking Hacks and Kitchen Essentials

A well-equipped kitchen can make meal preparation easier and more enjoyable when managing DGP. Here are some helpful tools:

- **Blender and Food Processor**: These appliances are lifesavers for puréed foods and smoothies.
- **Slow Cooker or Instant Pot**: These appliances allow for slow cooking and tenderizing of meats and vegetables, making them easier to digest.
- **Low-Fiber or Pre-Chopped Vegetables**: Opt for pre-chopped or frozen vegetables to save time and minimize prep work.
- **Low-Sodium Broths**: These broths add flavor to soups and other dishes without adding unnecessary salt.

Cooking Hacks

- **Cooking in Small Batches**: This ensures you have fresh, easily digestible meals readily available.
- **Thicken Soups and Smoothies**: Utilize low-fat yogurt, avocado, or nut butter to add thickness and creaminess without compromising digestion.
- **Freeze Portions**: Prepare larger batches of puréed foods or soups and freeze them in individual portions for quick and easy meals.

Remember, you're not alone in managing DGP. With the right tools, resources, and a positive attitude, you can live a fulfilling life despite this condition. This chapter equips you with the knowledge and strategies to not only manage DGP but also thrive and enjoy the journey.

DGP 14-Day Meal Plan

This two-week meal plan offers a variety of delicious and easy-to-digest options for breakfast, lunch, dinner, and snacks, all designed to be friendly for those with diabetic gastroparesis. Remember, portion sizes are crucial, so adjust as needed.

Day 1:
Breakfast: Smoothie with Protein Powder
Lunch: Vegetable Soup
Dinner: Baked Fish with Lemon and Herbs
Snack: Greek Yogurt Parfait

Day 2:
Breakfast: Scrambled Eggs with Spinach and Cheese
Lunch: Turkey Sandwich
Dinner: Chicken and Vegetable Stir-Fry
Snack: Banana Ice Cream

Day 3:
Breakfast: Quinoa Rice and Shine with Pureed Fruits
Lunch: Egg Salad Lettuce Wraps
Dinner: Spaghetti Squash with Marinara Sauce
Snack: Celery and Peanut Butter

Day 4:
Breakfast: Baked Omelet Muffins
Lunch: Tuna Salad
Dinner: Cauliflower Soup
Snack: Chia Pudding

Day 5:
Breakfast: Hot Cereal with Nut Butter
Lunch: Chicken Caesar Lite
Dinner: Zucchini Bake
Snack: Trail Mix

Day 6:
Breakfast: Breakfast Burrito
Lunch: Hummus Veggie Wrap
Dinner: Baked Sweet Potato with Cinnamon and Butter
Snack: Berries and Cream

Day 7:
Breakfast: Cottage Cheese and Berries
Lunch: Gazpacho
Dinner: Quinoa Salad with Roasted Vegetables
Snack: Almond and Date Energy Balls

Day 8:
Breakfast: Smoothie with Protein Powder
Lunch: Vegetable Soup
Dinner: Chicken Noodle Soup
Snack: Almond and Date Energy Balls

Day 9:
Breakfast: Scrambled Eggs with Spinach and Cheese
Lunch: Turkey Sandwich
Dinner: Quinoa Salad with Roasted Vegetables
Snack: Cucumber and Hummus

Day 10:
Breakfast: Baked Omelet Muffins
Lunch: Tuna Salad
Dinner: Delicious Simple Soup
Snack: Chia Pudding

Day 11:
Breakfast: Hot Cereal with Nut Butter
Lunch: Chicken Caesar Lite
Dinner: Baked Fish with Lemon and Herbs
Snack: Trail Mix

Day 12:
Breakfast: Breakfast Burrito
Lunch: Hummus Veggie Wrap
Dinner: Spaghetti Squash with Marinara Sauce
Snack: Berries and Cream

Day 13:
Breakfast: Stuffed Potato
Lunch: Mushroom Chicken Marsala
Dinner: Chicken and Vegetable Stir-Fry
Snack: Cottage Cheese Fruit Bowl

Day 14:
Breakfast: Veggie Scramble
Lunch: Gazpacho
Dinner: Egg Salad with Whole Grain Crackers
Snack: Berries and Cream

Conclusion

You did it! You flipped the script on diabetic gastroparesis. This book wasn't just about recipes; it was your personal rebellion against blandness, a middle finger to feeling limited. Now, the kitchen is yours again, a playground of flavors waiting to be explored.

These recipes are your weapons, but trust us, they're way more fun than peashooters. Imagine a creamy avocado smoothie that tastes like a tropical vacation, or a velvety soup that warms your soul from the inside out. Picture decadent desserts that don't leave you feeling like a ticking time bomb.

This isn't just about food, though. It's about reclaiming a piece of yourself. It's about late-night fridge raids with your bestie over a bowl of protein-packed goodness, or quiet mornings where a sunshine-in-a-glass smoothie jumpstarts your day. It's about taking back those stolen moments of joy, proving that even with a curveball like DGP, you can still have a life that's bursting with flavor.

So, from the bottom of our hearts, thank you for choosing this book. Thank you for taking a chance on a new way of eating. You're an inspiration, a warrior against blandness, a champion of flavor. We know you can turn this diagnosis into an epic culinary adventure.

Now, get out there and conquer your kitchen! Experiment, tweak, and most importantly, have fun. This journey might have bumps along the way, but with these recipes as your guide, you'll be a master chef of deliciousness in no time. Remember, every bite is a victory, a celebration of your strength and resilience. Here's to good food, good times, and a future filled with flavor. Bon appétit, and fight on!

Conversion Charts and Measurement Guides

Understanding measurements is key to following recipes accurately. This guide provides helpful conversions to ensure your diabetic gastroparesis meals turn out perfectly.

Household Measurements to Metric Equivalents: Here's a quick reference for converting common household measurements you might find in recipes to their metric equivalents:

- 1 cup (cup) = 240 milliliters (mL)
- ½ cup (½ cup) = 120 milliliters (mL)
- ¼ cup (¼ cup) = 60 milliliters (mL)
- ⅓ cup (⅓ cup) = 80 milliliters (mL)
- 1 tablespoon (Tbsp) = 15 milliliters (mL)
- 1 teaspoon (tsp) = 5 milliliters (mL)

Milliliters (mL) to Fluid Ounces (fl oz) Conversion:
If you find a recipe with measurements in milliliters (mL) but prefer using fluid ounces (fl oz), this conversion helps:

- 1 milliliter (mL) = 0.0338 fluid ounces (fl oz)

- Multiply the number of milliliters by 0.0338 to find the equivalent amount in fluid ounces.

Grams (g) to Ounces (oz) Conversion:
Similarly, for recipes using grams (g) and you'd like to convert them to ounces (oz):

- 1 gram (g) = 0.0353 ounces (oz)
- Multiply the number of grams by 0.0353 to find the equivalent amount in ounces.

Tips:
* Invest in measuring cups and spoons with metric markings for easy conversion.
* Many kitchen appliances, like blenders and food processors, come with measurement markings on their containers.
* Online conversion calculators are readily available for quick reference during recipe preparation.

Remember, these are general conversions. Always double-check the recipe's instructions for specific measurement preferences. With a little practice, converting measurements will become second nature, allowing you to whip up delicious and healthy diabetic gastroparesis meals with confidence!

Weekly Meal Journal

WEEK: _____

Sunday
- Breakfast
- Lunch
- Dinner
- Snacks

Monday
- Breakfast
- Lunch
- Dinner
- Snacks

Tuesday
- Breakfast
- Lunch
- Dinner
- Snacks

Wednesday
- Breakfast
- Lunch
- Dinner
- Snacks

Thursday
- Breakfast
- Lunch
- Dinner
- Snacks

Friday
- Breakfast
- Lunch
- Dinner
- Snacks

Saturday
- Breakfast
- Lunch
- Dinner
- Snacks

NOTES:

Weekly Meal Journal

WEEK: _____

Sunday
Breakfast
Lunch
Dinner
Snacks

Monday
Breakfast
Lunch
Dinner
Snacks

Tuesday
Breakfast
Lunch
Dinner
Snacks

Wednesday
Breakfast
Lunch
Dinner
Snacks

Thursday
Breakfast
Lunch
Dinner
Snacks

Friday
Breakfast
Lunch
Dinner
Snacks

Saturday
Breakfast
Lunch
Dinner
Snacks

NOTES:

Weekly Meal Journal

WEEK: _____

Sunday
- Breakfast
- Lunch
- Dinner
- Snacks

Monday
- Breakfast
- Lunch
- Dinner
- Snacks

Tuesday
- Breakfast
- Lunch
- Dinner
- Snacks

Wednesday
- Breakfast
- Lunch
- Dinner
- Snacks

Thursday
- Breakfast
- Lunch
- Dinner
- Snacks

Friday
- Breakfast
- Lunch
- Dinner
- Snacks

Saturday
- Breakfast
- Lunch
- Dinner
- Snacks

NOTES:

Weekly Meal Journal

WEEK: _____

Sunday
- Breakfast
- Lunch
- Dinner
- Snacks

Monday
- Breakfast
- Lunch
- Dinner
- Snacks

Tuesday
- Breakfast
- Lunch
- Dinner
- Snacks

Wednesday
- Breakfast
- Lunch
- Dinner
- Snacks

Thursday
- Breakfast
- Lunch
- Dinner
- Snacks

Friday
- Breakfast
- Lunch
- Dinner
- Snacks

Saturday
- Breakfast
- Lunch
- Dinner
- Snacks

NOTES:

Weekly Meal Journal

WEEK: _____

Sunday
- Breakfast
- Lunch
- Dinner
- Snacks

Monday
- Breakfast
- Lunch
- Dinner
- Snacks

Tuesday
- Breakfast
- Lunch
- Dinner
- Snacks

Wednesday
- Breakfast
- Lunch
- Dinner
- Snacks

Thursday
- Breakfast
- Lunch
- Dinner
- Snacks

Friday
- Breakfast
- Lunch
- Dinner
- Snacks

Saturday
- Breakfast
- Lunch
- Dinner
- Snacks

NOTES:

Weekly Meal Journal

WEEK: _____

Sunday
- Breakfast
- Lunch
- Dinner
- Snacks

Monday
- Breakfast
- Lunch
- Dinner
- Snacks

Tuesday
- Breakfast
- Lunch
- Dinner
- Snacks

Wednesday
- Breakfast
- Lunch
- Dinner
- Snacks

Thursday
- Breakfast
- Lunch
- Dinner
- Snacks

Friday
- Breakfast
- Lunch
- Dinner
- Snacks

Saturday
- Breakfast
- Lunch
- Dinner
- Snacks

NOTES:

Weekly Meal Journal

WEEK: _____

Sunday
- Breakfast
- Lunch
- Dinner
- Snacks

Monday
- Breakfast
- Lunch
- Dinner
- Snacks

Tuesday
- Breakfast
- Lunch
- Dinner
- Snacks

Wednesday
- Breakfast
- Lunch
- Dinner
- Snacks

Thursday
- Breakfast
- Lunch
- Dinner
- Snacks

Friday
- Breakfast
- Lunch
- Dinner
- Snacks

Saturday
- Breakfast
- Lunch
- Dinner
- Snacks

NOTES:

Weekly Meal Journal

WEEK: _____

Sunday
- Breakfast
- Lunch
- Dinner
- Snacks

Monday
- Breakfast
- Lunch
- Dinner
- Snacks

Tuesday
- Breakfast
- Lunch
- Dinner
- Snacks

Wednesday
- Breakfast
- Lunch
- Dinner
- Snacks

Thursday
- Breakfast
- Lunch
- Dinner
- Snacks

Friday
- Breakfast
- Lunch
- Dinner
- Snacks

Saturday
- Breakfast
- Lunch
- Dinner
- Snacks

NOTES:

Weekly Meal Journal

WEEK: ....

Sunday
- Breakfast
- Lunch
- Dinner
- Snacks

Monday
- Breakfast
- Lunch
- Dinner
- Snacks

Tuesday
- Breakfast
- Lunch
- Dinner
- Snacks

Wednesday
- Breakfast
- Lunch
- Dinner
- Snacks

Thursday
- Breakfast
- Lunch
- Dinner
- Snacks

Friday
- Breakfast
- Lunch
- Dinner
- Snacks

Saturday
- Breakfast
- Lunch
- Dinner
- Snacks

NOTES:

Weekly Meal Journal

WEEK: _____

Sunday
- Breakfast
- Lunch
- Dinner
- Snacks

Monday
- Breakfast
- Lunch
- Dinner
- Snacks

Tuesday
- Breakfast
- Lunch
- Dinner
- Snacks

Wednesday
- Breakfast
- Lunch
- Dinner
- Snacks

Thursday
- Breakfast
- Lunch
- Dinner
- Snacks

Friday
- Breakfast
- Lunch
- Dinner
- Snacks

Saturday
- Breakfast
- Lunch
- Dinner
- Snacks

NOTES:

Weekly Meal Journal

WEEK: _____

Sunday
Breakfast
Lunch
Dinner
Snacks

Monday
Breakfast
Lunch
Dinner
Snacks

Tuesday
Breakfast
Lunch
Dinner
Snacks

Wednesday
Breakfast
Lunch
Dinner
Snacks

Thursday
Breakfast
Lunch
Dinner
Snacks

Friday
Breakfast
Lunch
Dinner
Snacks

Saturday
Breakfast
Lunch
Dinner
Snacks

NOTES:

Weekly Meal Journal

WEEK: ....

Sunday
Breakfast ....
Lunch ....
Dinner ....
Snacks ....

Monday
Breakfast ....
Lunch ....
Dinner ....
Snacks ....

Tuesday
Breakfast ....
Lunch ....
Dinner ....
Snacks ....

Wednesday
Breakfast ....
Lunch ....
Dinner ....
Snacks ....

Thursday
Breakfast ....
Lunch ....
Dinner ....
Snacks ....

Friday
Breakfast ....
Lunch ....
Dinner ....
Snacks ....

Saturday
Breakfast ....
Lunch ....
Dinner ....
Snacks ....

NOTES:
....
....
....

Weekly Meal Journal

WEEK: _____

Sunday
- Breakfast
- Lunch
- Dinner
- Snacks

Monday
- Breakfast
- Lunch
- Dinner
- Snacks

Tuesday
- Breakfast
- Lunch
- Dinner
- Snacks

Wednesday
- Breakfast
- Lunch
- Dinner
- Snacks

Thursday
- Breakfast
- Lunch
- Dinner
- Snacks

Friday
- Breakfast
- Lunch
- Dinner
- Snacks

Saturday
- Breakfast
- Lunch
- Dinner
- Snacks

NOTES:

Weekly Meal Journal

WEEK: ....

Sunday
- Breakfast
- Lunch
- Dinner
- Snacks

Monday
- Breakfast
- Lunch
- Dinner
- Snacks

Tuesday
- Breakfast
- Lunch
- Dinner
- Snacks

Wednesday
- Breakfast
- Lunch
- Dinner
- Snacks

Thursday
- Breakfast
- Lunch
- Dinner
- Snacks

Friday
- Breakfast
- Lunch
- Dinner
- Snacks

Saturday
- Breakfast
- Lunch
- Dinner
- Snacks

NOTES:

Weekly Meal Journal

WEEK: ....

Sunday
Breakfast
Lunch
Dinner
Snacks

Monday
Breakfast
Lunch
Dinner
Snacks

Tuesday
Breakfast
Lunch
Dinner
Snacks

Wednesday
Breakfast
Lunch
Dinner
Snacks

Thursday
Breakfast
Lunch
Dinner
Snacks

Friday
Breakfast
Lunch
Dinner
Snacks

Saturday
Breakfast
Lunch
Dinner
Snacks

NOTES:

Weekly Meal Journal

WEEK: ....

Sunday
- Breakfast
- Lunch
- Dinner
- Snacks

Monday
- Breakfast
- Lunch
- Dinner
- Snacks

Tuesday
- Breakfast
- Lunch
- Dinner
- Snacks

Wednesday
- Breakfast
- Lunch
- Dinner
- Snacks

Thursday
- Breakfast
- Lunch
- Dinner
- Snacks

Friday
- Breakfast
- Lunch
- Dinner
- Snacks

Saturday
- Breakfast
- Lunch
- Dinner
- Snacks

NOTES:
....
....
....
....

Weekly Meal Journal

WEEK: ....

Sunday
- Breakfast
- Lunch
- Dinner
- Snacks

Monday
- Breakfast
- Lunch
- Dinner
- Snacks

Tuesday
- Breakfast
- Lunch
- Dinner
- Snacks

Wednesday
- Breakfast
- Lunch
- Dinner
- Snacks

Thursday
- Breakfast
- Lunch
- Dinner
- Snacks

Friday
- Breakfast
- Lunch
- Dinner
- Snacks

Saturday
- Breakfast
- Lunch
- Dinner
- Snacks

NOTES:

Weekly Meal Journal

WEEK: ....

Sunday
- Breakfast
- Lunch
- Dinner
- Snacks

Monday
- Breakfast
- Lunch
- Dinner
- Snacks

Tuesday
- Breakfast
- Lunch
- Dinner
- Snacks

Wednesday
- Breakfast
- Lunch
- Dinner
- Snacks

Thursday
- Breakfast
- Lunch
- Dinner
- Snacks

Friday
- Breakfast
- Lunch
- Dinner
- Snacks

Saturday
- Breakfast
- Lunch
- Dinner
- Snacks

NOTES:

Weekly Meal Journal

WEEK: ....

Sunday
- Breakfast
- Lunch
- Dinner
- Snacks

Monday
- Breakfast
- Lunch
- Dinner
- Snacks

Tuesday
- Breakfast
- Lunch
- Dinner
- Snacks

Wednesday
- Breakfast
- Lunch
- Dinner
- Snacks

Thursday
- Breakfast
- Lunch
- Dinner
- Snacks

Friday
- Breakfast
- Lunch
- Dinner
- Snacks

Saturday
- Breakfast
- Lunch
- Dinner
- Snacks

NOTES:

Weekly Meal Journal

WEEK: _____

Sunday
- Breakfast
- Lunch
- Dinner
- Snacks

Monday
- Breakfast
- Lunch
- Dinner
- Snacks

Tuesday
- Breakfast
- Lunch
- Dinner
- Snacks

Wednesday
- Breakfast
- Lunch
- Dinner
- Snacks

Thursday
- Breakfast
- Lunch
- Dinner
- Snacks

Friday
- Breakfast
- Lunch
- Dinner
- Snacks

Saturday
- Breakfast
- Lunch
- Dinner
- Snacks

NOTES:

Weekly Meal Journal

WEEK: ....

Sunday
- Breakfast
- Lunch
- Dinner
- Snacks

Monday
- Breakfast
- Lunch
- Dinner
- Snacks

Tuesday
- Breakfast
- Lunch
- Dinner
- Snacks

Wednesday
- Breakfast
- Lunch
- Dinner
- Snacks

Thursday
- Breakfast
- Lunch
- Dinner
- Snacks

Friday
- Breakfast
- Lunch
- Dinner
- Snacks

Saturday
- Breakfast
- Lunch
- Dinner
- Snacks

NOTES:

www.ingramcontent.com/pod-product-compliance
Lightning Source LLC
Chambersburg PA
CBHW071054240526
45471CB00015B/1936